Body Area Networks

Safety, Security, and Sustainability

Body area networks (BANs) are networks of wireless sensors and medical devices embedded in clothing, worn on or implanted in the body, and have the potential to revolutionize healthcare by enabling pervasive healthcare. However, due to their critical applications affecting human health, challenges arise when designing them to ensure they are safe for the user, sustainable without requiring frequent battery replacements, and secure from interference and malicious attacks. This book lays the foundations of how BANs can be redesigned from a cyber-physical systems perspective (CPS) to overcome these issues. Introducing cutting-edge theoretical and practical techniques, and taking into account the unique environment-coupled characteristics of BANs, the book examines how we can re-imagine the design of safe, secure, and sustainable BANs. It features real-world case studies, with suggestions for further investigation and project ideas, making it invaluable for anyone involved in pervasive and mobile healthcare, telemedicine, medical apps, and other cyber-physical systems.

SANDEEP KUMAR SHRINATH GUPTA is Professor, Founding Chair of the Computer Engineering Graduate Program, and Director of the IMPACT Lab, School of Computing, Informatics, and Decision Systems Engineering (SCIDSE), Arizona State University, USA.

TRIDIB MUKHERJEE is a Research Scientist at Xerox Research Centre, Bangalore, India.

KRISHNA KUMAR VENKATASUBRAMANIAN is an Assistant Professor at the Worcester Polytechnic Institute, Massachusetts, USA.

Body Area Networks

Safety, Security, and Sustainability

SANDEEP K. S. GUPTA
Arizona State University, USA

TRIDIB MUKHERJEE
Xerox Research Centre, India

KRISHNA KUMAR VENKATASUBRAMANIAN
Worcester Polytechnic Institute, USA

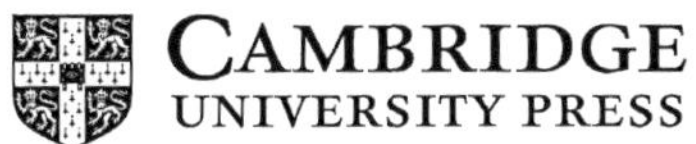
CAMBRIDGE
UNIVERSITY PRESS

CAMBRIDGE UNIVERSITY PRESS
Cambridge, New York, Melbourne, Madrid, Cape Town,
Singapore, São Paulo, Delhi, Mexico City

Cambridge University Press
The Edinburgh Building, Cambridge CB2 8RU, UK

Published in the United States of America by Cambridge University Press, New York

www.cambridge.org
Information on this title: www.cambridge.org/9781107021020

First published 2013

Printed and bound in the United Kingdom by the MPG Books Group

A catalog record for this publication is available from the British Library

Library of Congress Cataloging in Publication data
Gupta, Sandeep K. S., 1966–
Body area networks : safety, security, and sustainability / SANDEEP K. S. GUPTA,
TRIDIB MUKHERJEE, KRISHNA KUMAR VENKATASUBRAMANIAN.
    pages   cm
Includes index.
ISBN 978-1-107-02102-0
1. Body area networks (Electronics)   I. Mukherjee, Tridib.
II. Venkatasubramanian, Krishna Kumar.   III. Title.
TK5103.35.G86   2013
610.285′468–dc23

2012042718

ISBN 978 1 107 02102 0 Hardback

To my mother and in loving memory of my father
Sandeep
To Trijoy
Tridib
To my parents
Krishna

Contents

Foreword by Celeste R. Fralick   *page* xi
Preface   xv
Acknowledgments   xvii

1 Introduction   1
   1.1 Pervasive healthcare   2
   1.2 Monitoring technologies   4
   1.3 Overview of the book   7
   1.4 Questions   8

2 Body area networks   9
   2.1 Architecture   10
      2.1.1 Hardware   10
      2.1.2 Network topology   11
      2.1.3 Communication technology   12
      2.1.4 Software   15
      2.1.5 Deployment   15
      2.1.6 The physical environment   15
      2.1.7 Energy source   15
   2.2 Applications   16
      2.2.1 Physiological monitoring   16
      2.2.2 The infusion-pump control system 20
   2.3 Middleware for a BAN-based pervasive health-monitoring system 22
   2.4 Questions   25

3 BAN models and requirements   26
   3.1 Principal requirements   27
      3.1.1 Safety   27
      3.1.2 Security   28
      3.1.3 Sustainability   29
   3.2 The cyber-physical nature of BANs   30
   3.3 Regulatory issues   33
      3.3.1 Medical-device regulation in the USA   33
      3.3.2 Medical-device regulation in the EU   35
      3.3.3 Medical-device regulation in Asia   35

4   **Safety**   36
    4.1   Safety approaches   37
        4.1.1   Perspectives of BAN safety   37
        4.1.2   Ensuring BAN safety   39
    4.2   Model-based engineering of BANs   40
        4.2.1   Safety-requirements analysis   41
        4.2.2   Model generation   41
        4.2.3   Analysis of safety   42
    4.3   Modeling cyber-physical systems   42
    4.4   Example: BAND-AiDe – BAN Design and Analysis Tool   44
        4.4.1   The BAND-AiDe modeling framework   44
        4.4.2   The BAND-AiDe analyzer   49
        4.4.3   Implementation   50
    4.5   Demonstrating design and analysis with BAND-AiDe   53
        4.5.1   Safety verification of a single wearable medical device   56
        4.5.2   Safety verification of a network of devices   58
    4.6   Formal models for BAN safety   60
    4.7   Future research problems   61
    4.8   Questions   62

5   **Security**   63
    5.1   The need for information security in BANs   64
    5.2   Securing a BAN as a cyber-physical system   65
        5.2.1   Securing BAN components   66
        5.2.2   Challenges for CPS-Sec solutions   66
        5.2.3   CPS-Sec solutions for BANs   67
    5.3   Traditional security solutions for BANs   68
        5.3.1   Application of traditional approaches to key distribution 68
    5.4   Physiological-signal-based key agreement (PSKA)   70
        5.4.1   Physiological signals: issues and properties   71
        5.4.2   PSKA protocol execution   73
        5.4.3   Security of PSKA   76
        5.4.4   PSKA prototype implementation   78
    5.5   Summary and future research problems   82
    5.6   Questions   83

6   **Sustainability**   84
    6.1   The energy perspective   84
        6.1.1   Energy storage   85
        6.1.2   Reducing the energy requirement   86
        6.1.3   Scavenging energy from different sources   87
    6.2   The equipment-recycling perspective   87
    6.3   Ensuring sustainability   87
    6.4   Sustainable BAN software-design methodology   89

	6.4.1	The physical plane	90
	6.4.2	BAN application	91
	6.4.3	The management plane	92
6.5	Power profiling		92
6.6	Architectural modeling		93
6.7	Analysis and design for sustainability		95
	6.7.1	Sustainability analysis	98
	6.7.2	Case-study design	100
6.8	Future research problems		102
6.9	Questions		103

7   Implementation of BANs — 104

7.1	Implementation		104
	7.1.1	The computation model of a sensor node	105
	7.1.2	The computation model of a base station	106
7.2	Programming paradigms		107
	7.2.1	Programming a sensor	107
	7.2.2	Programming a base station	108
7.3	Common implementation issues		108
	7.3.1	Avoid floating-point operations	109
	7.3.2	Variable reuse and concurrency conflicts	111
	7.3.3	Storage management	112
	7.3.4	Distinction between tasks and event handlers	112
	7.3.5	Real-time considerations	112
	7.3.6	Debugging strategies	113
7.4	Diverse sensor platforms		113
7.5	Choosing the best platform		114
7.6	Automatic code generation		115
7.7	Data repositories		117
7.8	Questions		117

8   Epilogue — 119

Glossary	121
Appendix: Publication venues, academic research groups, and funding agencies	127
References	128
Index	138

Foreword

Over the last decade, the looming collision of the healthcare domain with a number of factors has led to a stark realization that change is urgently required. One may see this change in political platforms and government reforms, but it is technology that has been – and will continue to be – a driving force for the improvement of healthcare.

Factors contributing to this collision in the healthcare domain include the often-documented fact that global aging (contributed largely by the "baby boomer" generation, those born between 1946 and 1964) has hastened the need for increased efficiencies and improved patient outcomes. People aged sixty years and older will comprise at least 21.8% of the population in 2050. Given chronic care expenditures (78% of healthcare costs) and global shortages in hospital beds, assisted living housing, and healthcare professionals, it has been widely acknowledged that the response needs to be swift and thorough. With the US gross domestic product predicted to be at least 25% healthcare-related by 2025, current healthcare costs simply cannot be maintained without causing significant negative impacts on economic and social indicators.

Concurrently, demands for electronic medical records (EMRs) and vast health-information exchanges – analogous to the overhaul of the banking industry that brought us ATMs and electronic banking – are increasing as the need for connectivity and mobility permeates society. Little tolerance remains for paper entries and the nearly 100,000 medical errors seen yearly in the USA alone. While many facilities have successfully embraced EMRs, the global adoption rate continues to be low. Efficiency tools such as Lean and Six Sigma have been used within healthcare facilities to reduce costs, with promising results, but with inconsistent application.

In its infancy telemedicine was not embraced by clinicians due to lack of reimbursement from government or private insurance, lack of strong evidence-based data tied to medical outcome, technology challenges, and lack of usability. Forty years later, telemedicine is being identified as a key to solving the impending onslaught of elders. Improvements of technology connectivity, infrastructure, and device interoperability have encouraged managed-care and government agencies to invest in studies of remote healthcare monitoring in a variety of clinical settings, with promising results. By connecting vital-sign body area sensors (e.g., blood-pressure monitors, glucose-level monitors, pulse oximeters, weight scales, peak-flow meters) to aggregate form-factor "managers" or "hubs" (e.g., computers, USB devices, smart phones, and purpose-built devices) patients can be remotely monitored to reduce office visits and unnecessary hospitalization, increase clinician efficiency, and provide healthier functioning of the chronically ill. Recently, telemedicine has had a profound impact on returning physically and/or mentally disabled war veterans, since leaving the safety and ease of their home compounds their anxiety about returning to civilian life.

As technology improves and Moore's law (transistor density doubles every 12–18 months) continues to prove true, simple point solutions within the healthcare domain are necessary but not sufficient to address healthcare costs and associated economic and social conundrums. The increase in computer processing speeds, hyperthreading, and multi-cores with ever-decreasing footprints have placed a large amount of computing power in the hands of the product developers as well as consumers. Features such as advanced vector floating-point operations, integrated graphics, and high-speed input/output (I/O) (combined with the decreasing cost of memory and mass storage) are hastening the implementation of real-time and predictive clinical and operational analytics, gesture recognition in neural rehabilitation, discrete sensor capture, and four-dimensional (4D) imaging. Network bandwidth improvement, servers capable of managing "big data," and the implementation of hardware virtualization are all contributing to this phenomenon. These hardware improvements – coupled with emerging software efficiencies – in innovative and networked devices and systems can positively impact patient outcomes and lower healthcare costs. Networked devices that are in, on, or around the body (i.e., body area networks or BANs) provide an exciting opportunity for the consumer or patient to take more responsibility for his/her own healthcare, bringing self-sufficiency and the possibility of revolutionary approaches to tackling global healthcare challenges.

With the advent of placing more and more sensors in the ecosystem, safety and security are paramount to user experience, clinical interpretation, and positive patient outcomes. Global regulatory and certification bodies oversee most aspects of safety; however, it is the modeling, design, experimental, and analytic testing acumen (discussed in Chapter 4) prior to formal clearance and approval that meet and exceed the requirements. These approaches are critical to ensuring that subsequent changes in hardware, software, and usage are unequivocally safe. Thorough verification and validation (even for a non-regulated medical product) are necessary to ensure we are testing the "right things right." That is inclusive of security as well – over 88,000 security breaches are occurring daily, with recent reports of medical-device malware and hospital-record breaches. Unique approaches (such as the physiological-signal-based key agreement detailed in Chapter 5), coupled with improvements to hardware and software security technology throughout the entire network, are critical for broad BAN acceptance and trust of sensor data.

Lastly, no product should be developed today without careful consideration of sustainability. Power harvesting from unique sources will allow BANs to be deployed with energy efficiency for reliable and user-friendly experiences (discussed in Chapter 6). Even frequent implanted battery changes (at intervals of 3–5 years) require more "patient-on-table" time, obvious risks notwithstanding. Thus, reducing energy needs through careful modeling and design methods can provide increased reliability and opportunities to analyze and design sustainable solutions.

In this book the reader shall discover a plethora of innovative guidance and solutions to BANs. BANs are a critical and technological response to increasing global healthcare challenges that embrace the very nature of the need: bring a systematic solution to the product developer and consumer for better patient accountability and outcomes. Gupta, Mukherjee, and Venkatasubramanian provide a critical and thorough assay of BANs, covering their architecture, models, and requirements, and enable the reader to invoke improved safety, security, and sustainability of BANs. With the congruence of aging populaces, rising healthcare costs, remote monitoring, EMRs, and advancing technology, it is now up to the reader to understand and implement BANs to positively change the future of global healthcare.

Celeste R. Fralick, MSE
Staff Architect and Principal Engineer
Intel Corporation

CELESTE R. FRALICK is currently a Staff Architect and Principal Engineer at Intel Corporation. Her technical oversight includes the embedded intelligent systems in the medical sector. Her unique expertise spans 32 years, including positions with Medtronic, Texas Instruments, and Fairchild Semiconductor. She was a key developer of Intel's initial biotechnology strategies, culminating in Intel's first regulated medical device. She has served on the Advisory Board for the Biodesign Institute, the Bioengineering Advisory Committee, and the College of Nursing's Healthcare Innovation and Clinical Trials Advisory Board at Arizona State University. She has also served on the Scientific Advisory Board for the World Nanotechnology Conference, as chair of the 2005 International Global Digital Healthcare conference, and as a board member for Arizona State University's WinTECH, MacroTechnology Works' Healthcare Innovation Program, She continues to be an Associate Editor with the *Journal of Biomedical Microdevices*, remains on the Board of Directors for the AZ Health-e Connection and the International Essential Tremor Foundation, and on iNEMI's TIG for Medical Device Components, and recently became a research faculty member for Health and Medicine in the International Institute of Analytics.

Preface

Over the last decade, developments in miniaturization and low-powered electronics have led to the development of wireless sensor networks (WSNs), which are computational systems with the ability not only to sense their environments, but also to process and communicate the data obtained using a wireless channel. This book focuses on a specific class of WSNs, called body area networks (BANs) (also known in the literature as body sensor networks), which are networks of wireless sensors worn on or implanted within the human body and have the potential to revolutionize healthcare by enabling anytime and anywhere health monitoring and actuation. Already a plethora of applications for BANs is being developed for a variety of settings in order to provide managed care both for chronic and for acute conditions. For example, BANs have been developed for monitoring soldiers on the battlefield, managing patients in forward locations in a disaster-hit region, emergency management, elder care, and rehabilitation purposes. However, in order for these applications to be viable in the long run, it is necessary to design BANs to be safe in terms of not causing harm to the users, sustainable without requiring frequent battery replacements, and secure from clandestine eavesdropping or interference. These are particularly challenging problems given the complexity of BANs and the limited computational and communication resources available at the devices/sensors in the BANs.

An important feature of BANs is that their constituent devices/sensors directly interact with their environment (i.e., the human body) in order to operate. This environment-coupled nature of BANs puts them within a new class of systems called cyber-physical systems (CPSes), which are systems featuring a tight combination of, and coordination between, the system's computational (e.g., sensors) and physical elements (e.g., the human body). This book explores how BANs can be designed from this CPS perspective. One needs to employ a model-based approach for designing BANs taking into account their environment-coupled nature. Specifically, the book focuses on three aspects of BANs:

- safety – ensuring that side-effects of operation on the environment (human body) are within desired limits
- sustainability – ensuring uninterrupted operation of the BAN
- security – ensuring authorized actions on the BAN

This book is organized into seven chapters. Chapter 1 focuses on providing the context for this work in terms of sensors, which form the basis of BANs. It provides an overview of using sensors for health-monitoring purposes, thus providing an overview of the origin and need for BANs. Chapter 2 delves deeper and provides a comprehensive overview of BANs and their principal components and properties. Chapter 3 then moves on to providing an overview of the principal approach we take to designing BANs – a model-based environment-coupled approach – together with associated issues such as regulatory issues.

After the introduction provided by the first three chapters, we move on to the core of the book that pertains to designing safe, secure, and sustainable BANs. Each of the next three chapters tackles one of these issues using a model-based environment-coupled approach, and provides a case-study demonstrating the working of the approach. Chapter 4 presents a model-based engineering approach to improve the safety of BANs. The chapter also provides a case-study featuring the safety-design and analysis tool called BAND-AiDe to study the thermal effects of sensor operation on the human body. Chapter 5 presents an environment-coupled approach to improve the security of BANs. A case-study utilizing physiological signals to enable key agreement between sensors is presented. Chapter 6 then moves to sustainability issues in BANs. Here, models of various BAN architectures and energy sources are used in conjunction to design sustainable BANs. We present a case-study that demonstrates the effectiveness of various energy-scavenging mechanisms in sustaining a health-monitoring BAN. Each of these three chapters also features open research questions.

Finally, Chapter 7 concludes the book with a summary of how to actually go about implementing a safe, secure, and sustainable BAN designed in the earlier chapters, including a discussion on a systematic methodology for choosing a platform that is most suited for a given application.

This book has been written with advanced courses and graduate-level seminars in mind. It will allow students to gain a conceptual appreciation of BANs in general and, more specifically, using the model-based environment-coupled design methodology for designing them. At the end of each chapter bar one, the book provides questions that are designed to induce a student to think about the contents of the chapter and find solutions. Additional material, including programming assignments and lecture slides, is available online at `http://impact.asu.edu/BANBook.html`. This book will also be of interest to people who are interested in the up and coming field of cyber-physical systems and want an overview of how to go about designing them. Additionally, practitioners in the applications area will find the book useful as a book on the new domain.

Acknowledgments

Throughout the writing of this book, many people have helped us; without them, this book would not have been possible. First and foremost we thank Ayan Banerjee for helping immensely with various aspects of the book, including contributions to formal analysis and synthesis of BANs as well as implementation of body sensor networks, organizing and proof-reading the book, and help with the figures and indexing. We are grateful to Celeste Fralick, of Intel Corp., for her insightful foreword and her comments on various aspects of the book from the perspective of her vast experience in technologies for healthcare. Many thanks are due to Paul Jones, of the US Food and Drug Administration, for his comments on regulatory aspects covered in the book. The quality of this book has been much improved by their comments and contributions. The authors are solely responsible for any remaining errors or omissions in the book.

Various past and current researchers of the IMPACT Lab at Arizona State University have collaborated with us on topics related to this book. We greatly appreciate their visionary work and dedication.

Our heartfelt thanks go to Dr. Phil Meyler, Publishing Director, Engineering, Mathematical and Physical Sciences at Cambridge University Press for encouraging us to write this book and to Mia Balashova, Publishing Assistant, Engineering who provided the needed level of support and encouragement to see this book through from conception to completion. Her periodic emails enquiring about the status of the book draft served as an important beacon to see this book safely ashore. We also thank all the people at Cambridge University Press who oversaw the copyediting process, and the entire crew of Cambridge University Press.

We thank our respective present and past employers, Arizona State University, Xerox Corp., the University of Pennsylvania, and Worcester Polytechnic Institute, for providing the working environment that made this book possible. We are grateful to the National Science Foundation (NSF) for support through programs such as Information Technology Research (ITR), CyberTrust (CT), and Smart Health and Wellbeing (SHB), and to the National Institutes of Health (NIH), Food and Drug Administration (FDA), Google Corp., and Intel Corp. for supporting our research in the areas related to this book. We also thank Byron Gillespie, of Intel Corp., for helping us garner financial support to develop pedagogical material for this book.

Last but not least, we thank our family members and friends who accepted the time away from them spent writing this book. Without their understanding and support, this book could never have been finished.

1 Introduction

A healthy populace is essential for societal prosperity and well-being. This makes healthcare a basic societal necessity. Most societies endeavor to provide it in some form, usually in an organized manner through a system of medical facilities that are either private or public, or both. The current mode of delivering care relies on the patient initiating the care-delivery process. Figure 1.1 illustrates this model. It is a four-step process and requires the patient to observe the presence of specific symptoms, and visit a caregiver, who then diagnoses the problem and provides a treatment. We call this the *traditional model of care delivery*. The principal characteristic of the traditional model is that it is reactive in nature. No action is taken to improve the patient's condition unless the patient initiates the process. A problem with this approach is that it is inherently defensive in nature in fighting illness. This is particularly problematic if the symptoms for the patient's ailments seem benign or manifest late in the progression of the disease.

Additionally, the traditional model has other problems as well, especially those associated with scale. The whole model of care was designed for a society where the number of people requiring care was a very small percentage of the population. However, with the dramatic demographic shift taking place in the world, especially that associated with aging, the traditional model of care delivery will be a huge bottleneck. Furthermore, the societal demographic shift is also producing one at the level of caregivers, leading to a dramatic decrease in the number of caregivers available in certain specialties [1]. This will most likely lead to dire shortages of healthcare personnel, and, if this situation is left unattended, could result in a drop in the quality of medical care and a substantial increase in healthcare costs [2, 3]. In summary, with the traditional model of care delivery in place, the healthcare system in most countries will (the US healthcare spending is projected by the Centers of Medicare and Medicaid to be 4.5 trillion by 2019 [4]) increasingly come under pressure as the average age of their population increases and the number of elderly people swells.

One of the ways of reversing this trend is by the introduction of automated pervasive health-monitoring technologies that can monitor a person's health and alert appropriate healthcare personnel in case of emergencies, thereby providing optimal care with minimal supervision. In response to this need, embedded computing devices such as smart phones, iPads®, and other personal electronic devices are being increasingly used to support health-related applications such as tracking calorie intake [5], weight control [6], pulse oximetry [7], and educational training for nurses [8]. Trends indicate a fast progression towards pervasive health-monitoring systems (PHMSes), where sensors

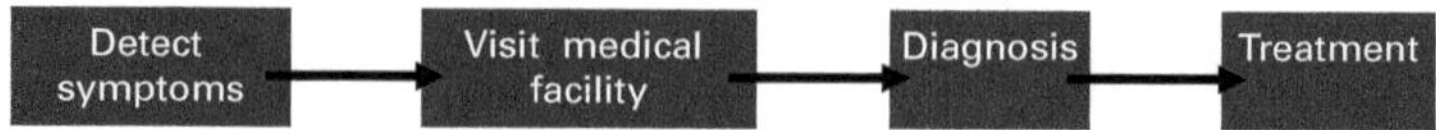

Figure 1.1   The traditional healthcare-delivery model.

are deployed on the human body to monitor environmental and physiological signals, a smart phone acts as a computation and communication hub, or base station, for these sensors, which gathers data and processes them to detect contexts, such as location, activities, or health emergencies, and a personal laptop uploads information to the cloud to form a history of health. With the smart phone being recently considered as a medical device [9], PHMSes are predicted to become critical infrastructures to support the health and well-being of the populace. *Pervasive healthcare* can play a major role in providing continuous care to patients, thereby altering the traditional care-delivery model into one that provides healthcare facilities to individuals anywhere and at any time. It uses large-scale deployment of sensing and communication (wired and wireless) technologies to monitor patients continuously. This allows it to deliver accurate health information to caregivers, thereby stimulating timely diagnosis and treatment for health problems.

1.1   Pervasive healthcare

Significant advances in communication and sensing technologies have led to the development of intelligent hand-held and wearable devices (such as smart phones, smart clothes, and smart apparel). Such devices provide a platform to implement a wide range of solutions for health-monitoring purposes. Examples include vital-signs-monitoring apps available on various smart phones. Further, their wearable or hand-held nature allows them to be present around the user at all times, making health monitoring a pervasive activity. We call such technologies that use pervasive computing capability for health management *pervasive healthcare systems.*

The health-monitoring capability of pervasive healthcare systems makes them ideal for many diverse applications [10], including the following. (1) *Telemedicine.* This provides the ability to monitor, diagnose, and treat patients anytime and anywhere. The automation brought about by the technology further reduces the chances of errors and enables timely treatment of patients by providing accurate, real-time, and complete health information to the caregivers. (2) *Lifestyle management.* Pervasive healthcare systems have the ability to provide personalized care by keeping track of a user's health in minute detail and providing the information as needed. For example, it can be used by people to improve their health by developing specialized meal and exercise plans. (3) *Data repositories.* Pervasive healthcare systems are designed to collect data from patients over long periods of time. These data are stored in an organized manner so that they can be studied by the patients' caregivers in order to provide better care. Such large data sets can be useful for studying issues such as the response to medicine, the demographics of people with specific ailments, possible improvements in the care, improvement in medicine, alternative treatments, and diagnosis.

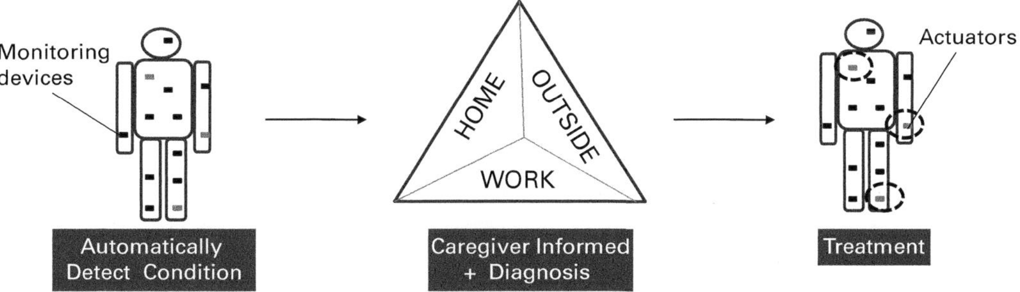

Figure 1.2   The envisioned healthcare-delivery model.

Pervasive healthcare systems by their very nature alter the traditional treatment model by making it more proactive. They provide a proactive patient-centric form of care (as opposed to the reactive caregiver-centric form of today's care), which permits health problems to be detected and responded to as soon as they occur. Now, the presence of an ailment will be detected way in advance before some or even any of the symptoms manifest themselves. This detection of the ailment will cause the information to be made available to the caregiver directly. No personal visit is required immediately. The caregiver analyzes the data, performs diagnosis, and specifies treatment for the user, which can be provided to the user through the use of actuation devices or may require the patient to visit the caregiver. An additional advantage of the pervasive monitoring system from the perspective of the caregivers is that a single caregiver can now manage a large number of patients. Further, this can be done without any time or space restrictions for either the caregiver or the patient. Figure 1.2 illustrates this newly envisioned healthcare-delivery model.

Conceptually, the model consists of three main planes. The model has been adapted from the one presented in [11]. Figure 1.3 illustrates the three planes. The three planes are the device plane, the data-access plane, and the knowledge plane. The *device plane* is used to collect medical data from patients and perform preliminary processing on it. It consists of a large number of medical devices that possess the capability to collect both physiological and ambient data from around the patients. The devices may be deployed on patients in both in-vivo and in-vitro manner. The data collected from the devices are handled by the *data-access plane*, which serves three purposes: (1) enabling the devices to interact seamlessly with one another; (2) providing facilities for organizing pre-processed health data from devices into a structured electronic format (also known as electronic patient records (EPRs), electronic health records (EHRs), or electronic medical records (EMRs)), and for their long-term storage; and (3) enabling device actuation as a treatment measure. The data-access plane also provides the infrastructure for managing the health data collected by the devices. Finally, the *knowledge plane* is used for reasoning on the data in the EPRs. Some of the features it can provide include detection of the occurrence of a medical emergency, the failure of a specific treatment procedure, and inconsistencies between the proposed diagnosis and the symptoms. This capability gives the caregivers feedback pertaining to their diagnoses and treatment,

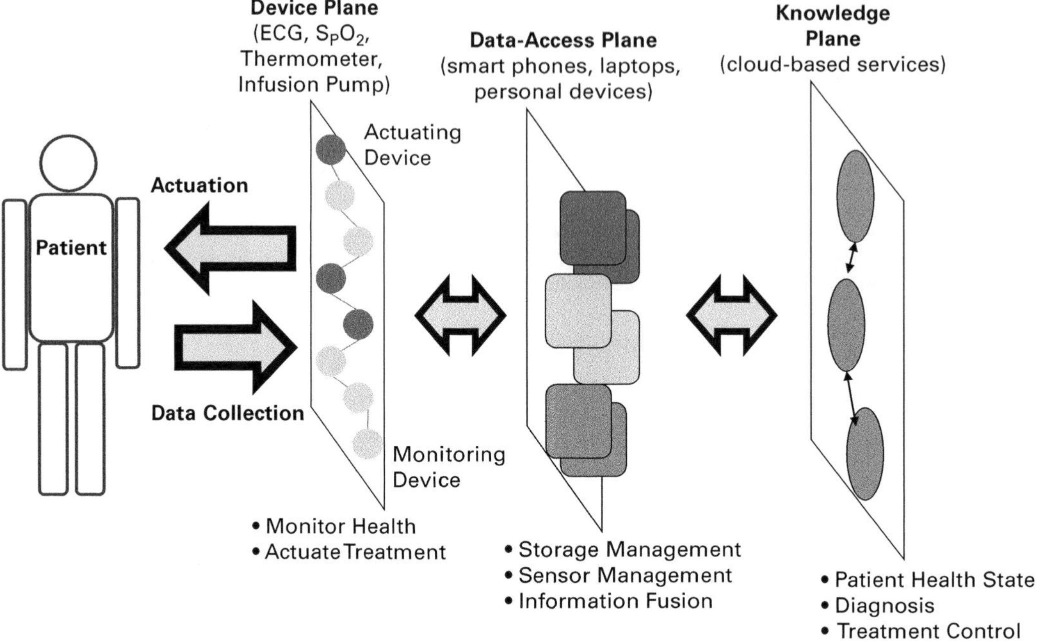

Figure 1.3   The pervasive healthcare model: conceptual view.

allowing them to make appropriate adjustments through the data-access plane. Recent initiatives by the US government have resulted in the Health Information Exchange (HIE) cooperative agreement program (`http://healthit.hhs.gov/portal/server.pt?open=512&objID=1488&mode=2`), which encourages exchange of health information between different healthcare facilities throughout the USA.

1.2   Monitoring technologies

One of the most pressing needs in modern medicine is to develop medical devices capable of providing continuous care (i.e., monitoring, decision support, and delivery of therapy). Such devices are expected to decrease healthcare costs by enabling alternatives such as home-based or ambulatory care. This allows caregivers to permanently have a detailed picture of the patient's health, enabling them to better tune the treatment provided. Such a system also makes possible real-time notification in the event of emergencies and providing first-responders with accurate and complete information about the patient's health.

These new-generation medical devices are usually cyber-physical in nature; that is, they are very tightly coupled with their environment (the human body). Further, since they are being designed for long-term monitoring purposes, they usually have a very small form factor with minimal power footprint, and use wireless communication technologies where possible. They have been designed to monitor a plethora of ailments,

Table 1.1 Prominent pervasive care systems

Pervasive care system	Sensor type	Purpose
SenseWear[a]	Wearable monolithic device	Physical-activity and sleep-behavior monitoring
Microcompaq[b]	Wearable monolithic device	Continuous monitoring of vital signs
UbiMon[c]	Wearable and implantable sensors	Capturing transient but life-threatening medical events
HealthGear[d]	Wearable sensors	Detecting sleep apnea
MyHeart[e]	Biomedical smart clothes	Monitoring/detecting cardiovascular diseases
CodeBlue[f]	Wearable sensors	Emergency care, disaster response, and stroke rehabilitation
Lifeshirt[g]	Wearable sensors	Continuous monitoring of vital signs
Ayushman[h]	Wearable sensors	Continuous monitoring of vital signs

[a] http://sensewear.bodymedia.com/
[b] http://www.welchallyn.com/
[c] http://www.doc.ic.ac.uk/vip/ubimon/home/index.html
[d] http://research.microsoft.com/~nuria/healthgear/healthgear.htm
[e] http://www.hitech-projects.com/euprojects/myheart/
[f] http://www.eecs.harvard.edu/~mdw/proj/codeblue/
[g] http://www.lifeshirt.com
[h] http://impact.asu.edu/Ayushman.html

such as cardiovascular diseases and neurological problems, rehabilitation, and general health, and for collecting meta-physiological-state information (sleep, awake, fatigue), circadian activity monitoring, extreme-environment medical monitoring (e.g., space), and sleep monitoring. The biomedical platforms developed in this regard can be broadly classified into three broad categories: (1) monolithic platform-based, (2) textile (fabric)-based, and (3) body-sensor-network-based. Some of the prominent health-monitoring BANs are listed in Table 1.1.

Monolithic platform-based solutions

Monolithic solutions consist of devices that are basically a micro-controller board used as a medical monitoring platform. Various (often custom-designed) physiological monitoring sensors (biosensors) are used to collect specific physiological parameters and transfer them to the board for signal processing and storage. The monitoring platform usually forwards the patient data to the back-end (hospital network) for storage. This is usually done via a wireless channel in order to ensure the patient's mobility. Such monolithic monitoring devices allow the monitoring of a diverse set of physiological signals such as the electrocardiogram (ECG), photoplethysmogram (PPG), electromyogram (EMG), galvanic skin response (GSR), skin temperature, and blood pressure (BP). Some of the prominent projects in this category include the LiveNet at MIT [12], AMON at the ETHZ [13], and LifeGuard at NASA Ames and Stanford [14]. Such systems, given their monolithic nature, are easy to manage; however, they possess minimal intelligence, and packing all the sensors with one board makes the entire setup bulky, with relatively large form factors affecting its usability.

Textile-based solutions

Textile-based medical monitoring platforms try to alleviate some of these problems by distributing the sensors over a fabric worn by a person, making them truly wearable health-monitoring systems. Textile-based platforms integrate biosensors into the fabric of the garment by using conductive fibers, which are knitted like regular yarn. The entire system is supplied by a centralized portable power source, which is a part of a micro-controller board that is used to collect, process, and possibly forward (to back-end entities, wirelessly) data from the sensors. No wireless module is required at the sensors since the fabric itself acts as a data-bus. As in the previous case, textile-based monitoring platforms enable the monitoring of a slew of physiological parameters such as the ECG, EMG, activity (accelerometer), PPG, skin temperature, GSR, BP, and body temperature. Some of them even have the ability to raise alarms if the physiological parameters go beyond preset thresholds [15]. The platforms typically differ in terms of the fibers used for knitting the garment (conductive and/or electrostrictive), the type of garment (vest or covering the entire upper body), and usability (washable, stretchable). Some of the prominent systems which use the textile-based approach to monitoring include MyHeart [16], Wealthy [15, 17, 18], MagIC [19], and SmartVest [20]. The systems also vary in terms of the available signal-processing capabilities, with respect to removing measurement artifacts, removing baseline noise from ECG signals, and individualized calibration of sensors. Textile-based systems have the advantages of being easier to use, and providing good signal quality and comfort. However, the dramatic shift in paradigm has made their adoption very slow. In [21], the authors posit that the principal reasons for this are the limited involvement from the stake-holders, the yet-to-be-proven clinical effectiveness of the technology, and the poor cost-to-benefit ratio for payers (insurance agencies) thus far, in terms of safety, security, and convenience.

Body-area-network-based solutions

The third category of next-generation medical devices are those which form a network on the person being monitored using a large number of low-capability computing platforms called sensors. These body sensor networks (BSNs) or body area networks (BANs) use tiny wireless-enabled processing units (often referred to as motes in the literature), which are usually interfaced with one or more custom-designed or off-the-shelf sensing modules, also called *motes*. The data from the sensing modules are collected by the mote, and forwarded wirelessly to a base station for long-term storage and processing. The motes equipped with a micro-controller can do limited amounts of processing, such as reducing motion artifacts and carrying out signal cleaning. The wireless channel used also varies with the platform used, with ZigBee, IEEE 802.15.4, and Bluetooth being the prominent technologies used. Some of the prominent applications based on BANs include CodeBlue at Harvard [22], the Alarm-Net platform at UVa [23],

Human++ [24], BASUMA [25], and HeartToGo [26]. The BAN-based systems have the advantage of being easy to deploy and manage. However, they do suffer from poor signal quality due to motion artifacts and from poor battery life, and the wireless channel used is susceptible to eavesdropping and jamming.

1.3　Overview of the book

In this book, we focus on the third type of continuous monitoring technologies available, i.e., body area networks. The principal idea is to ensure that BANs do not cause potential hazard to the human body from interruptions in, and side-effects of, their operation. For example, in a cardiac-care scenario with a BAN made of heart-function monitors (ECG, PPG sensors) and actuators (pacemakers), the potential hazards of operation include battery exhaustion (this interrupts the BAN's operation), initiation of unauthorized and untimely actuation (shocks) by replaying old commands (i.e., triggering unauthorized actions), and unwarranted electromagnetic interference from nearby electronic devices such as mp3 players inducing effects on long-term BAN operations. Consequently, the focus of this book is on how BANs can be designed in order to make them more safe, secure, and energy-wise sustainable for long-term operation. The emphasis is placed on software-engineering aspects of BANs.

The software-design methodology that is considered in this book is that of *model-based engineering* as shown in Figure 1.4. In this methodology, the given BAN system and its interaction with the human body and the environment (discussed in Chapter 2) are first represented using mathematical abstractions or models (Chapter 3). These models can be behavioral models that represent the operation of the BAN using transfer functions (Chapters 4 and 6), formal models that represent the system using finite-state machines (Chapters 4 and 6), hybrid systems, which model the cooperation of the embedded systems with the human physiology (Chapters 4 and 6), or feature-based

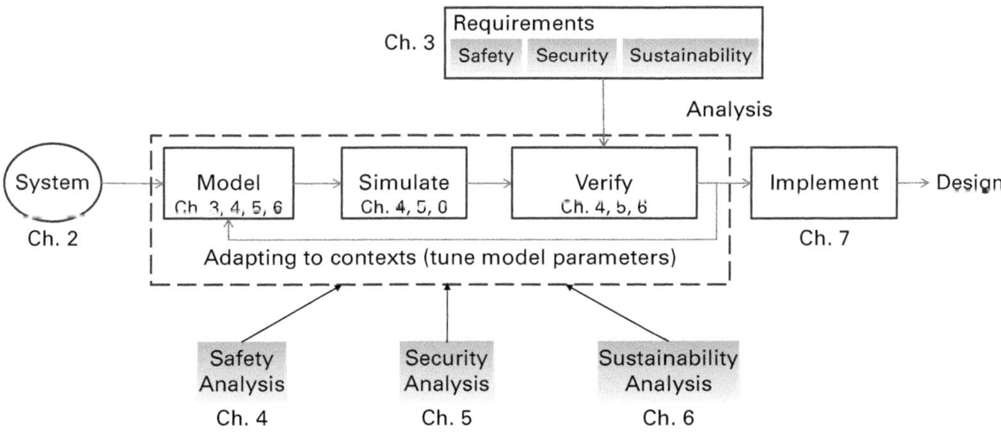

Figure 1.4　Model-based environmentally coupled solutions for BAN design.

representations obtained using signal-processing algorithms (Chapter 5). The models are then simulated, whereby the model parameters are mathematically manipulated in order to obtain the system behavior in terms of system properties. The system properties are then checked against the safety, security, and sustainability requirements (Chapter 3) to check for their violation. If there are violations, then the models are adapted to the environmental context, which includes the physiological state of the BAN user. The adaptation procedure typically involves tuning the model parameters or changing thresholds in the signal-processing algorithms. This procedure, also known as model-based analysis, is discussed in detail for each of the BAN requirements of safety (Chapter 4), security (Chapter 5), and sustainability (Chapter 6). The output of the model-based analysis phase is a BAN model that is verified against requirements. The next stage is the implementation of the model, which is handled by the design phase. The design phase is discussed in Chapter 7, where several automatic code-generation tools are described.

1.4 Questions

1. What are the advantages and disadvantages of the traditional healthcare model as described in Section 1?
2. Think of three potential applications for pervasive healthcare systems apart from the applications described in this chapter. Give as much detail as possible, including design diagrams.
3. One of the advantages of using pervasive healthcare systems is the automated population of electronic patient records (EPRs). These have slowly come to replace paper-based records in care facilities and afford many advantages. What are the advantages of EPR systems over paper-based records, and what, if any, are the potential disadvantages?
4. Imagine a hospice or elderly-care facility with about 10 patients being cared for. There is one medical team responsible for the health of all the patients, consisting of a primary-care provider, a geriatrics specialist, and a couple of nurses. Design a health-monitoring system for such a facility that can monitor patients continuously and provide the information to the care-providers using the technologies (one or more) described in this chapter. Discuss the potential performance, scalability, and usability of the system designed.

2   Body area networks

A body area network (BAN) is a network consisting of a heterogeneous set of *nodes* that can sense, actuate, compute, and communicate with each other through a multi-hop wireless channel. A BAN collects, processes, and stores physiological (such as electrocardiogram (ECG) and blood pressure), activity (such as walking, running, and sleeping), and environmental (such as ambient temperature, humidity, and presence of allergens) parameters from the host's body and its immediate surroundings; and can even actuate treatment (such as drug delivery), on the basis of the data collected. BANs can be very useful in assisting medical professionals to make informed decisions about the course of the patient's treatment by providing them with continuous information about the patient's condition.

BANs belong to a much more generic class of device networks called wireless sensor networks (WSNs) [27]. BANs evolved from WSNs through a series of intermediate steps whereby first the WSN concept was applied to personal devices such as laptops, phones, cameras, and printers. Such networks are called personal area networks (PANs) [28], or wireless PANs (WPANs) [28]. From WPANs evolved BANs in which medical devices, such as pulse oximeters, and personal computing or auxiliary devices such as smart phones and retina prostheses [29, 30] were networked through the wireless channel and worn on the body. Devices were also implanted, such as pacemakers, which communicate through the body to an outside controller. In a hospital setting, BANs are networked with other in-hospital medical devices such as Holter monitors and medical data recorders to form medical device networks (MDNs) [31] for post-operative or intensive-care-unit (ICU) patient monitoring.

Sensors form the essential basis of a BAN and come in different forms. Essentially sensors in BANs may have one or more of the following properties.

- They may be *heterogeneous* in terms of capabilities, and are designed to be *unobtrusive* to the host. Consequently, individual sensors in a BAN may have very *limited* form factor, power source, memory, computation, and communication capabilities, compared with generic sensor nodes, thus requiring BANs to employ a large number of nodes in order to collect patient health data in a reliable and fault-tolerant manner.
- They may be *implantable or wearable* in nature, implanted sensors are subject to more stringent requirements with respect to safety, security, and sustainability than do wearable ones.
- They may be designed to *measure multiple stimuli* from their environment (the human body).

- They may be designed to *survive extreme conditions* such as variation in temperature and the presence of water or saline [32].
- They may be *powered using scavenged energy* sources such as body movements, body heat production, flexible solar cells and biofuels such as blood glucose [32].

For example, implantable pacemakers need to operate in the presence of saline body fluids and may be operated using energy scavenged from body heat [33].

Each BAN has a controlling entity called the *base station*, which collects and processes data for the BAN. All the sensors in the BAN communicate the data they collect to the base station at regular intervals. BANs can vary in size from a network of a few nodes to a large network with a few hundred. Systems with upward of 150 sensors have been designed [34]. It has been suggested in [35] that a large number of low-quality sensors can perform the task of monitoring as effectively as a few high-quality sensors, while at the same time being less intrusive. Consequently, we assume that BANs with hundreds of sensors are feasible. Needless to say, BANs have many diverse applications, including sports health management, home-based healthcare for the elderly, and post-operative care.

2.1   Architecture

A BAN consists of a network of computing units that are used to perform context-aware ubiquitous operations to aid monitoring and autonomous actuation applications in healthcare, and for performance monitoring and giving feedback in military, leisure, and sports applications.

The nodes in a BAN are of varied capabilities; however, they can be broadly classified into two categories: (1) *sensor nodes*, which are implanted or wearable medical devices or simply low-capability wireless computing platforms interfaced with sensors and actuators (e.g., a PPG sensor interfaced with TelosB motes); and (2) *base-station* nodes, which have higher computational and communication capabilities (e.g., smart phones) than the worker nodes, and are used for disseminating information to and collecting information from the worker nodes. The base station controls the entire BAN and can reach every node in it in a single hop. It has significantly higher computational and communication capabilities than do the sensors, therefore all sensors send their data to it for processing. Note that, unlike in traditional wireless sensor network applications where there is limited control over the sensor networks after deployment, the BAN is a fairly controlled system, being under the supervision of the patient or medical personnel at all times. IEEE Task Group 6 (TG6) (`http://ieee802.org/15/pub/TG6.html`) has defined the standard architectures of a BAN. According to the standards the prominent characteristics of a BAN architecture can be summarized as follows.

2.1.1   Hardware

Sensors in a BAN are heterogeneous with respect to hardware configuration. With recent advances in embedded-systems research a plethora of small-scale computing units, radios, and storage devices can be implemented. Most of these are suitable candidates for BAN hardware. According to IEEE TG6, the hardware components of the BAN may be (1) a general-purpose sensor (e.g., TelosB motes, `http://www.xbow.com/`, in which a low-power micro-controller is interfaced with several sensors such as humidity, temperature, and light sensors), (2) a medical device (e.g., a pulse-oximeter device for monitoring the pulse rate of an individual, which consists of an LED array, a photodetector, a micro-controller, and a radio for communication purposes), (3) data collectors or aggregators, such as a bedside monitor or an image collector for a pill camera, (4) a controller or tuner, such as an infusion-pump controller, or (5) a gateway or access point, which can be a smart phone.

With regard to general-purpose sensing, several commercial BAN platforms have been proposed to provide the computation, communication, and storage backbone for the sensors. The processors that are extensively used in such platforms are MSP430 from Texas Instruments, xScale or Atom^{TM} from Intel®, ATMEGA 128 from Atmel®, and the ARM® processor. Also field-programmable-gate-array (FPGA)-based sensor nodes or application-specific-integrated-circuit (ASIC) components have been proposed for application-specific implementations. Further, hybrid platforms whereby different types of processors are integrated in the same board are being considered for better distribution of computation. In such cases, an FPGA might be interfaced with an Intel Atom® processor such that the computationally intensive signal-processing task can be delegated to the fast dedicated FPGA, while data-collection and -storage tasks can be performed by the Intel Atom®. Apart from general-purpose sensing, platforms for sensing and processing specific signals such as electrocardiograms and photoplethysmograms have been developed. Special attention to their easy wearability, implantability, and unobtrusiveness has yielded a plethora of flexible sensing devices such as ECG patches (`http://www2.imec.be/`), nanosensors (`http://www.nanosensors.com/`), and smart clothing (`http://www.crunchwear.com/`). Research in flexible electronics has further boosted wearable- or implanted-sensor design.

In the base station, the smart phones use the ARM or the Intel Atom processor, and are more sophisticated than the sensors.

2.1.2   Network topology

BANs consist of two types of computing units: (1) *sensor nodes*, which have a low processing capability; and (2) the *base station*, which is a high-end computing device such as a cell-phone or a PDA. In a BAN the computing units communicate with each other through a wireless channel, since wires running between sensors in a BAN would make it obtrusive. The sensor communication is assumed to be reliable, and each sensor is time synchronized, using several schemes that are based on packet-arrival time [36, 37]. Each node in a BAN has a set of neighboring nodes with which it can communicate through a one-hop wireless link (indicated by the communication range in Figure 2.1). Three network topologies have been recommended by IEEE TG6, as shown in Figure 2.2. Figure 2.2(a) shows the star topology, where each node has a one-hop wireless link to the base station. Multi-hop routing from the nodes to the base station

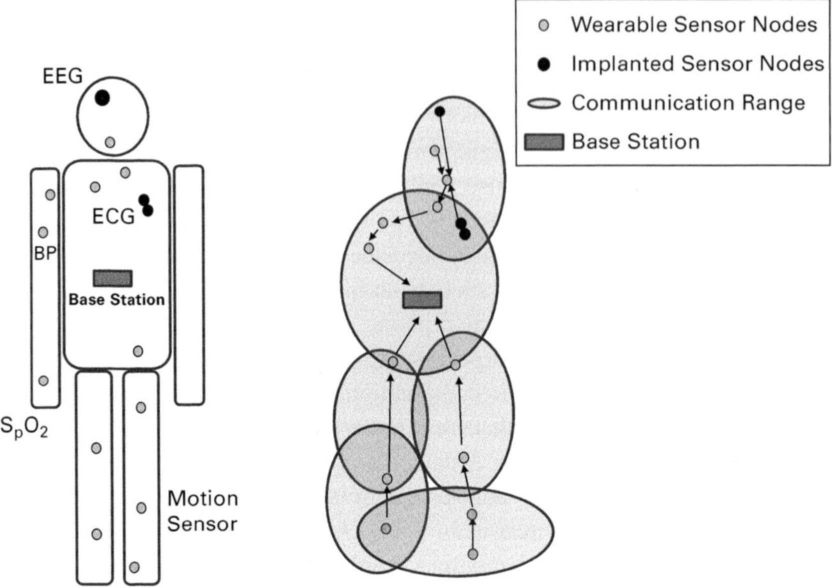

Figure 2.1   A body area network.

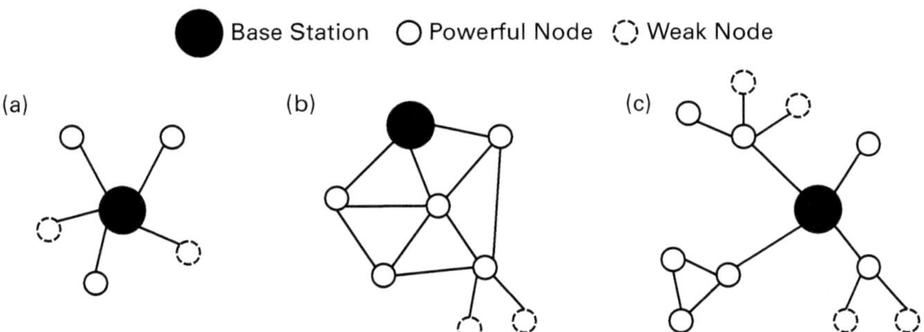

Figure 2.2   BAN network topologies recommended by IEEE TG6: (a) star topology, (b) mesh topology, and (c) hybrid topology.

is also recommended in the mesh topology shown in Figure 2.2(b). A combination of single-hop access to the base station for powerful nodes and multi-hop access for weaker nodes is employed, with the base station at the root collecting the data from all the sensor nodes [38], in the hybrid topology shown in Figure 2.2(c).

2.1.3   Communication technology

Several communication technologies have been proposed for BANs, which vary in range, power consumption, frequency of transmission, and form factor. The communication infrastructures for BANs have a similar layered structure to the OSI stack. As shown in Figure 2.3, the BAN communication protocol stack has five layers: (1) the

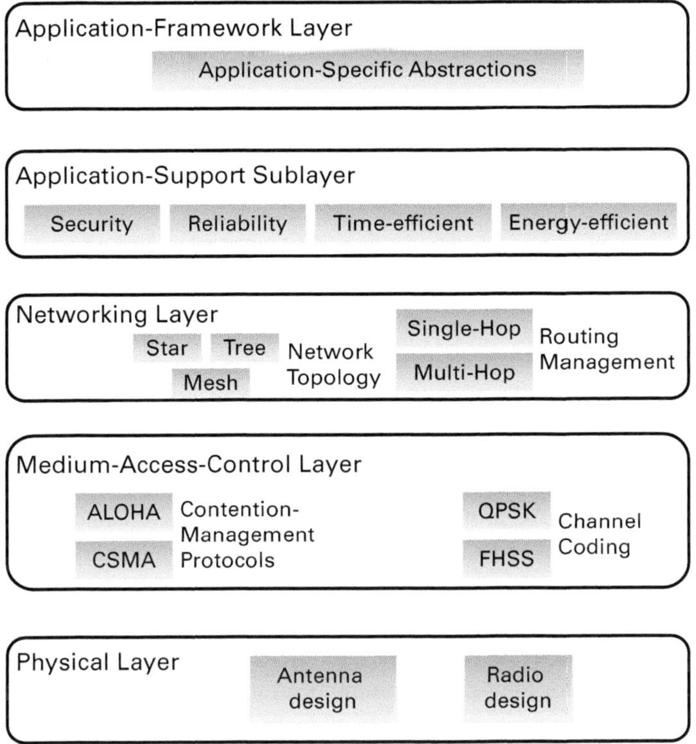

Figure 2.3   The protocol stack of a body area network.

physical layer, which deals with the antenna and radio hardware; (2) the medium-access-control (MAC) layer, which deals with channel access and contention management; (3) the network layer, which deals with routing management and reliable data transfer; (4) the application-support sublayer, which deals with applications such as securing the communication infrastructure; and (5) the application framework, which provides abstractions of the basic functionalities of the radio to any application.

Table 2.1 gives a list of the currently available radio technologies along with the IEEE TG6 recommendations. The characteristic of the communication technology depends on several factors.

- **Antenna design**. The quality of reception and transmission of data in the BAN depends largely on the design of the antenna. Since the form factor of sensor nodes in the BAN is constrained for easy wearability, the size of the antenna typically is very small. In some sensor nodes, such as Mica2 (`http://xbow.com`), the antenna is a quarter-wave dipole antenna that juts out from the PCB. However, in more current versions of the sensor nodes, such as in TelosB, BSN v3, Shimmer, and iMote2, the antenna is embedded in the PCB, where an inverted-F antenna, a miniaturized surface mount antenna, a chip antenna, and a full version of the surface mount antenna are used respectively. Owing to the antenna size the reception quality, measured using the packet-drop-ratio (PDR) metric, is affected. For example, at the same transmission

Table 2.1 Radio standards

	ZigBee	6lowPAN	Bluetooth low power	IEEE TG6 recommendation
Frequency	2.4 GHz	868/915 MHz	2.4 GHz	1 THz
Form factor	length 80 mm, width 26 mm, height 8.5 mm	12.7 mm × 25.4 mm × 3.5 mm	13.4 mm × 25.8 mm × 2 mm	No specific recommendation
Speed	250 kbps	250 kbps	3 Mbps	1 Gbps
Range	70 m	15 m	1–100 m	10 m
MAC protocol	CSMA-CA	QPSK	FHSS	
Power	2.5–100 mW	1 mW	75–90 mW	

power levels, the BSN v3 node has a very much lower PDR than that of the Imote2 node, which has the same antenna design.

- **MAC protocol.** The MAC protocol ensures that the wireless channel is accessed without contention and reliable data transfer is achieved. The principal types of radios used in BANs are listed in Table 2.1. The ZigBee radio is used for mesh networking and is particularly suitable for BAN multi-hop communication. The channel-contention policy used by ZigBee is carrier-sense multiple-access-collision avoidance (CSMA-CA), and is suitable for long-range communication with periodic data transfer. Often individual medical devices are interfaced to the smart phone through Bluetooth, which is suitable for short-range master–slave connection and intermittent transfer of data. Bluetooth uses the frequency-hopping spread-spectrum (FHSS) MAC protocol to resolve contention. However, such radio standards consume considerable amounts of power and are often not suitable for long-term or in-vivo operation. Hence, researchers have considered developing low-power radio standards such as 6lowPAN (`http://6lowpan.net`) and Bluetooth low power, which consume considerably less power.

- **Wireless channel.** The sensors in the BAN use the wireless channel to transfer data to the base station. The wireless channel is prone to errors such as random bit errors, burst errors, and fading errors [38–40]. Several different channel models have been considered for BAN communication, where path loss is modeled as Ricean or Rayleigh. However, since the sensors are around the human body and are confined within a smaller area, it is near-field communication (NFC) and the fading is of small scale [41]. Hence, a log-normal channel model fits better for BANs [41]. Over the years, researchers have also considered using the human body as the communication channel. IEEE TG6 has also provided the standards for channel models of the human body, namely biochannels. Further, using the human body as a channel reduces overhearing and hence improves security. However, safety issues such as radiation safety and thermal safety pose an important challenge in using the human body as the communication channel.

Note that in Table 2.1 IEEE TG6 recommends the usage of the 1-THz frequency band for BAN transmission. This recommendation is made keeping in mind the high interference in the most commonly used 2.4-GHz band, which causes high packet-drop rates.

2.1.4 Software

The BAN has two classes of software for programming the sensor and the base station. For the sensor, generally an event-driven programming paradigm is followed, whereby computation is scheduled on occurrence of an event. TinyOS is such an event-driven operating system, and is most commonly used for sensors. For the base station, there are three popular types of software used for smart phones: Android, which is open source, iOS, solely for programming iPhone by Apple, and Windows SilverLight.

2.1.5 Deployment

The sensors in the BAN are either worn on or implanted within the human body. The exact placement of sensors on or within the human body depends on the application. (e.g., fingertip pulse oximeters (www.smithsoem.com) are worn on the index finger). Further, recent research endeavors have networked the sensors in the BAN with car sensors to provide a car area network (CAN). Use of a BAN in automotive contexts has been shown to increase the safety of the driver by providing early feedback on fatigue. With the advent of social media such as Facebook, MySpace, and Google+, researchers have also investigated the combined usage of BAN and social media to facilitate easy sharing of health data and faster diagnosis [42].

2.1.6 The physical environment

The physical environment is the BAN deployment environment (generally the human body). The operation of the sensor nodes in the BAN is inherently coupled with the environment through sensing or actuation or through side-effects of the computing on the environment (e.g., heat dissipation).

2.1.7 Energy source

The sensors and base station of the BAN have to be wireless devices in order to facilitate user mobility. Hence, the primary power sources for these devices are batteries. The lifetime of the BAN devices is thus limited by the battery capacity. For designing sustainable BANs it is important to use the battery in an efficient way. This requires a BAN designer to understand the load characteristics of the battery as it ages. This section provides a survey on the characteristics of contemporary battery technology.

A battery is primarily a means of storage of electrical energy. Batteries can be broadly classified into two groups: (1) re-chargeable, which can be re-charged upon full discharge and reused; and (2) un-chargeable, which can be used only once and cannot be recharged. Typically, for smart-phone devices, which serve as the base station for the BAN, the batteries are re-chargeable, while for sensor devices both types are used, e.g., TelosB (`xbow.com`) sensors need battery replacements, while the shimmer sensors (`shimmer-research.info`), use re-chargeable batteries. A re-chargeable battery is characterized by five key properties.

- **Cycle life**. One cycle life of a battery is a discharge from full charge to full discharge and a return to full charge again. The battery capacity is often measured by the number of cycle lives it can provide before the peak voltage drops.
- **Fast charging time**. There are several methodologies to charge a battery. Typically a control circuitry is used to rapidly charge the batteries without damaging the cells' elements. Most such chargers have a cooling fan to help keep the temperature of the cells under control. Other existing types of charging are through USB and pulse chargers. The specification of a battery includes the fast charging time, which essentially lists the time taken to charge from zero to full charge using the control circuitry.
- **Overcharge tolerance**. Batteries charged without using the control circuitry can be subject to overcharge. Poles can get reversed if batteries are overcharged. Typically three levels of overcharge tolerance are reported – low, medium, and high.
- **Self-discharge rate**. When not used, the battery slowly drains its charge due to inefficiencies in its design, which gives rise to internal resistance.
- **Gravimetric energy density**. This is a term used for the amount of energy stored in a given system or region of space per unit volume.

2.2   Applications

BANs are used for a variety of applications including patient monitoring, sports monitoring, entertainment, and medical actuation. We discuss the processing and communication requirements in a BAN using two examples of physiological monitoring and medical control systems.

2.2.1   Physiological monitoring

In a physiological-monitoring application, the sensor in the BAN senses physiological signals such as the electrocardiogram (ECG) and the photoplethysmogram (PPG). Physiological signals have an underlying periodic nature, which BAN sensors can utilize to achieve energy-efficient sensing. Such underlying characteristics are complex and can be learned using models, as we shall discuss for two specific signals, namely the ECG and PPG.

Electrocardiograms capture the electrical pulses emitted due to the functioning of the heart. As shown in Figure 2.4, a single beat of an ECG consists of P, Q, R, S, and T waves, with a U wave present in some cases. The Q, R, and S waves are often jointly considered as a QRS complex. The shape, amplitude, and relative locations of the constituent waves are key features of an ECG, referred to as *morphology features*. The distance between two consecutive R peaks is called the R–R interval, and its reciprocal gives the instantaneous heart rate. The R–R interval typically varies over time, and this

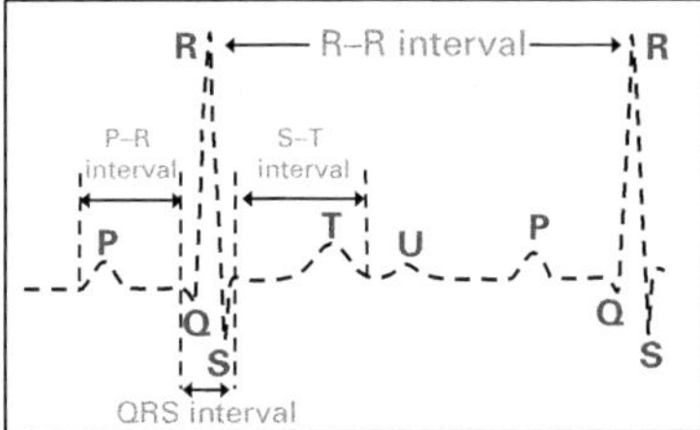

Figure 2.4   Morphology features of an ECG beat. A beat is comprised of P, Q, R, S, and T waves, with a U wave present in some cases.

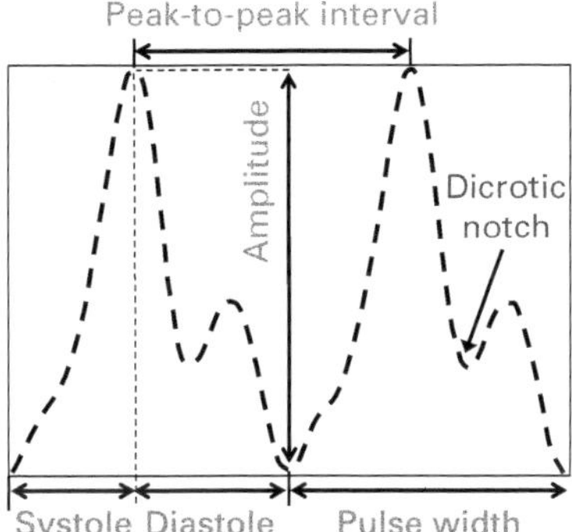

Figure 2.5   Salient features of a PPG pulse.

variation is described using temporal features such as the mean and standard deviation of the heart rate, and spectral features such as the low-frequency/high-frequency (LF/HF) ratio [43]. We refer to these features as *inter-beat features.*

Several mathematical models of the ECG have been proposed in the literature, of which we discuss the ECGSYN model [43]. In ECGSYN, the inter-beat features of the ECG (the mean and standard deviation of the heart rate and the LF/HF ratio) are modeled using three parameters: HR_{mean}, HR_{std}, and LF/HF ratio, respectively. For the morphology features, each wave (P, Q, R, S, and T) is represented by three parameters $(a, b,$ and $\theta)$, which determine its height, width, and distance to the R peak, respectively.

A typical PPG waveform contains a high-frequency component, called the pulsatile component, superimposed on a low-frequency baseline variation. The fundamental frequency of the pulsatile component depends on the heart rate and is generally around 1 Hz. The baseline variation is due to respiration, thermoregulation, and other physiological factors [44]. Most diagnostic applications that are based on PPG filter out the baseline variation and use only the pulsatile component [45]. Hence, we focus only on the pulsatile component of PPG.

Each pulse of the PPG signal, as shown in Figure 2.5, contains a rising edge corresponding to the systole (contraction of ventricles) and a falling edge corresponding to the diastole (relaxation of ventricles). These edges are hence referred to as the *systolic edge* and *diastolic edge*, respectively. The diastolic edge often has a notch, called the dicrotic notch, which is indicative of healthy arteries [44]. A single PPG pulse is characterized by its height, width, and shape. These are called the morphology features of the PPG, and are expected to remain fairly constant over short time scales for a given person [46]. The temporal characteristics of the PPG are studied using the peak-to-peak intervals among pulses. These intervals have been shown to correspond directly to the inter-peak intervals of the ECG [47], and hence can be characterized using well-known ECG inter-beat features [43]. These include temporal features such as the mean and standard deviation of the heart rate and frequency-domain features such as the LF/HF ratio.

The blood-pumping action of the heart has been modeled using the analogy of electrical circuits with resistive, capacitive, and inductive elements. These models are called windkessel models [48], and are extensively used to model blood-pressure variation in human body. The windkessel model provides a differential-equation model for the PPG signal, whose constant coefficients vary from one person to another and have to be learned. These differential equations can then be solved to obtain a time-series representation of the PPG.

These models of the physiological signals are used for efficient sensing of physiological signals as described in the following section.

Processing for energy-efficient data collection

In the generative-model-based resource-efficient-monitoring (GeM-REM) technique, the physiological signal is divided into three categories: (1) normal, when the temporal and morphological features of the signal do not change; (2) varying, when only the temporal features vary; and (3) abnormal, when both the temporal and the morphological signals vary. In the normal case, the signal is represented using the generative model at the base station, and no feature information is communicated. In the varying case, only the temporal features that change are communicated to the base station, instead of the actual signal samples, and the new temporal features are used in the generative model to regenerate the signal. In the abnormal case, all the signal samples are communicated back to the base station.

The idea of the generative-model-based technique is to reduce power-hungry communication to a minimum and increase the burden on low-power computation in order to achieve energy efficiency. In order to achieve this, it imposes very complex signal-processing requirements on the sensors. The processing requirements for a sensor to execute the model-based data collection technique for ECG are the following.

1. **Scaling.** The amplitude of the sensed ECG signal is highly dependent on the sensor hardware and the ECG lead configuration. To ensure an accurate comparison between the sensed data and the model data, they must both be converted to a common, device-independent scale. This is achieved by linearly scaling each signal to a maximum of 1.2 mV and a minimum of −0.4 mV.
2. **Filtering.** The sensed ECG is typically noisy, and must be filtered to extract the underlying signal. For extracting the QRS complex, a passband of 5–12 Hz is required, which is achieved by cascading lowpass and highpass filters with cutoff

frequencies of 5 Hz and 12 Hz, respectively. For low computational overhead, a finite-impulse-response (FIR) filter design of six taps and order 32 is used.

3. **Peak detection.** Measuring ECG features such as R–R intervals and the width of the QRS complex requires detecting Q, R, and S peaks. In order to perform this peak detection at low computational overhead, a lightweight QRS-peak-detection algorithm (see Algorithm 2.1) is used. This algorithm detects all the positive and negative peaks in a signal, and then imposes a relative threshold on the amplitude to qualify peaks as Q, R, and S. Further, false positives are reduced by imposing conditions that are based on the previous peak detected. For example, for a negative peak to be declared an S peak, the previous peak must be an R peak.

Once the pre-processing has been completed, the sensed ECG is compared with the signal generated by the model. Such a comparison is performed in two ways.

Feature-based comparison. In this approach, a set of features is extracted from both signals and their values are compared. We use this approach for the inter-beat features (the mean and standard deviation of the heart rate, and the LF/HF ratio) since they can be calculated from the sensed ECG at low computational cost. The mean and standard deviation of the heart rate are obtained by calculating the mean and standard deviation of a set of 30 consecutive R–R intervals. To optimize computation speed and power consumption, we developed an efficient TinyOS implementation for a fast Fourier transform

```
For each incoming data sample x[i]
    if (x[i] > MAX) Set MAX = x[i]
    if (x[i] < MIN) Set MIN = x[i]

    if (Looking for upward peak)
        if (x[i] < MAX) Mark x[i - 1] as PossiblePeak
        if (x[i] < (MAX - thresholdUp))
            Mark latest PossiblePeak as RealPeak
            if (magnitude(RealPeak) > thresholdR)
                Mark peak as R peak
            Start Looking for downward peak
    else      // looking for downward peak

        if (x[i] > MIN) Mark x[i - 1] as PossiblePeak
        if (x[i] > (MIN + thresholdDown))
            Mark latest PossiblePeak as RealPeak
            if ((magnitude(RealPeak) > thresholdQ)
                    AND (PreviousPeak is S))
                Mark peak as Q peak
            if ((magnitude(RealPeak) > thresholdS)
                    AND (PreviousPeak is R))
                Mark peak as S peak
            Start Looking for upward peak
```

Algorithm 2.1 The QRS detection algorithm used in the GeM-REM sensor module.

(FFT) for LF/HF-ratio computation. Once these calculations have been completed, the feature values are compared with the model parameter values HR_{mean}, HR_{std}, and LF/HF ratio, respectively.

Direct signal comparison. Calculating the morphology features involves complex curve fitting and is not feasible for computationally limited sensors. Hence, we use the direct signal-comparison approach for the ECG morphology. A sample, representative beat, referred to as MeanBeat, is obtained by averaging 10 consecutive beats of the sensed ECG. On the other hand, we use our lightweight ECGSYN implementation to generate a sample ECG beat, referred to as ModelBeat. The ModelBeat and MeanBeat are aligned by superimposing the respective R peaks, and the fit is compared using a mean-square error approach. The mean-square metric is chosen since it captures the shape as well as the amplitude of the Q, R, and S waves. Since generating the ModelBeat was found to be computationally expensive, it is performed only when the morphology parameter values are updated. The generated ModelBeat is then stored in memory for future use.

2.2.2   The infusion-pump control system

The infusion-pump control system is shown in Figure 2.6. The target open-loop system, the infusion-pump actuation module, which infuses drugs into the human body, has two types of inputs: (1) **programmed infusion rate**, namely the pump administers a constant infusion rate until this is changed; and (2) **bolus request**, namely a request for drug infusion from the patient, which causes a step rise in infusion rate for a given amount of time. The bolus request can be a random perturbation to the open-loop system.

The control algorithm for the infusion pump varies the programmed infusion rate of the pump to maintain a given concentration of the drug in the blood. The drug

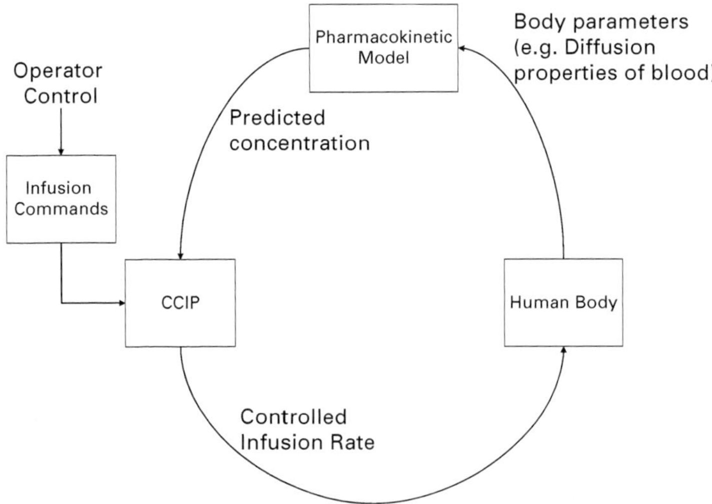

Figure 2.6   The infusion-pump control system.

concentration to maintain is given as the **reference input** to the control system. The control algorithm receives feedback from the human physiology. The feedback is obtained from a mathematical model representing the drug diffusion process in the human body, also called a pharmacokinetic model. This model predicts the future drug concentration due to the current infusion rate administered by the pump. The predicted drug concentration depends on the previous history of infusion, the current infusion rate, and the diffusion coefficients of the human body. The control algorithm takes the reference and the predicted drug concentration as input and computes the future infusion rate of the pump that is required in order to maintain the reference drug concentration in the blood.

Let us assume that the infusion pump has safety-verified software. According to the infusion-pump safety criteria as listed in the generic infusion-pump project [49], the infusion rate should not exceed $x\%$ of a preset value. However, this safety criterion does not correspond directly to patient safety. Further, when the medical device operates in a control loop with the human body as a feedback the drug concentration in the blood can become unstable and reach unacceptably high values even if the infusion rate remains within $x\%$ of the preset value, hence hampering patient safety. Simulations on a Simulink model of the infusion pump developed by an IMPACT Lab volunteer at the FDA confirms such patient safety violations. The parameters for the pump and the pharmacokinetic model were obtained from a case study on anesthesia infusion [50]. Figure 2.7(a) shows the infusion rate and the drug concentration in the blood over time for anesthesia infusion. From Figure 2.7(a) it can be seen that the infusion rate over time has significant **overshoot and undershoot** before it reaches a stable point. Further, significant amount of time, the **settling time**, is required for the drug concentration in the blood to reach the reference level set by the operator. A large settling time may lead to a delay in the therapeutic effect of the drug. In the case of mission-critical operations such as drug infusion to prevent cardiac arrest [51], a short settling time is essential in order to provide therapeutic effects within a window of opportunity.

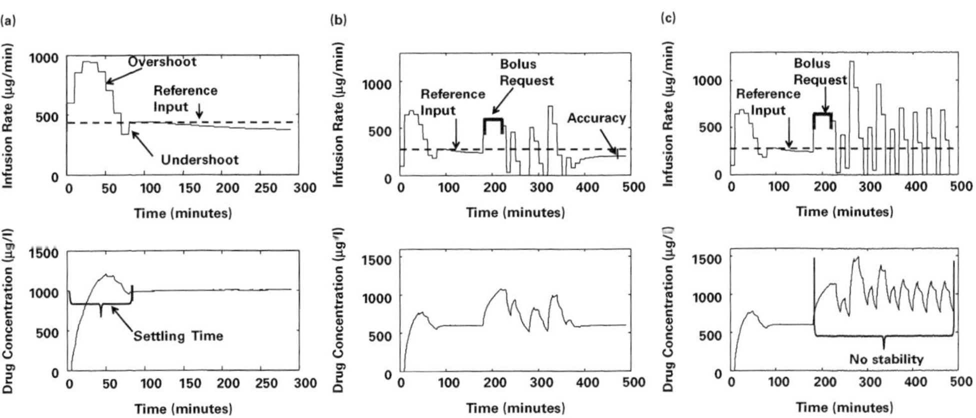

Figure 2.7 Anesthesia pump simulation with no bolus and at different levels of bolus showing overshoot, settling time, stable, and unstable behavior. Bolus administration is indicated by dark bold lines: (a) without bolus, (b) bolus at 600 µg/min, and (c) bolus at 650 µg/min.

Given these computation requirements from various BAN applications, we next discuss the resources provided by BANs for implementation.

2.3   Middleware for a BAN-based pervasive health-monitoring system

A pervasive health-monitoring system (PHMS) consists of a BAN with physiological sensors recording parameters such as the ECG and EMG as well as environmental signals such as temperature and humidity at the lowest level, and sensor management, data management, location management, and several other services at higher levels. The operation of a PHMS is characterized by dynamic changes in the user context [52], e.g., change in user location from home to outdoors for a jog or to a hospital in the case of a medical emergency (Figure 2.8). Such changes in context affect the operation of every subcomponent of a PHMS. To illustrate this claim, let us consider the example of

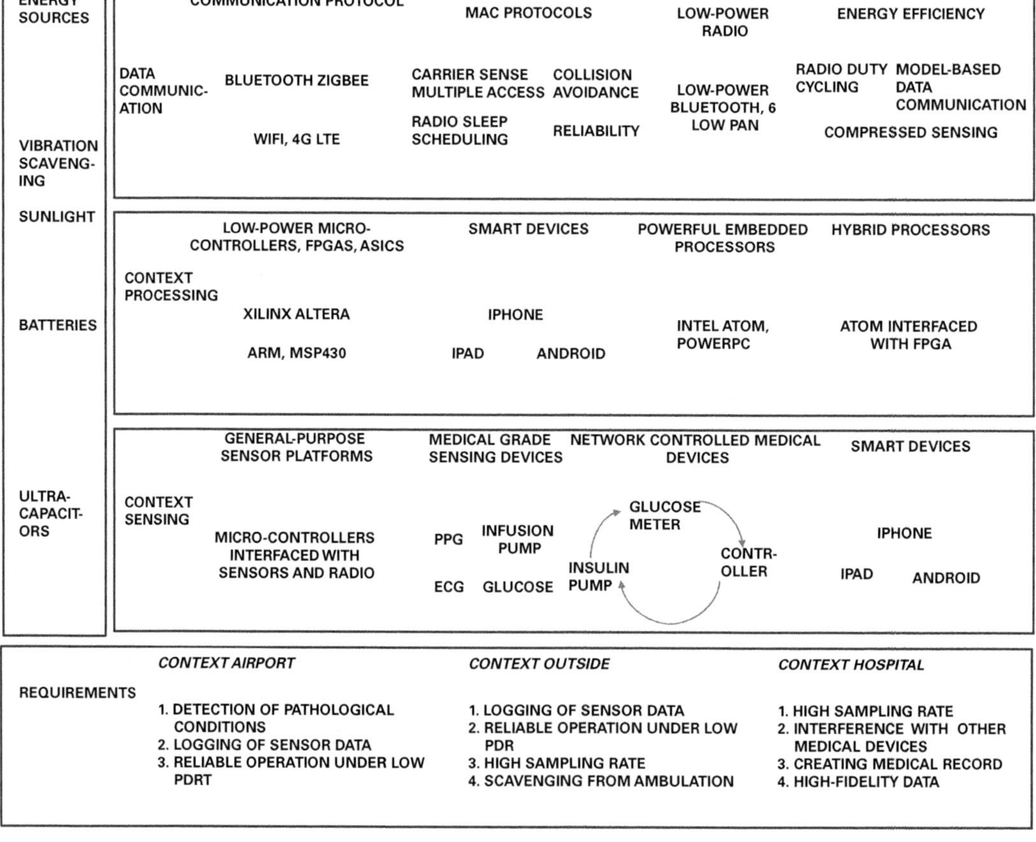

Figure 2.8   A PHMS in different contexts with varied requirements. The basic layers of PHMS have several design options for a designer. Choosing the right set of alternatives to match the system requirements is a challenging problem.

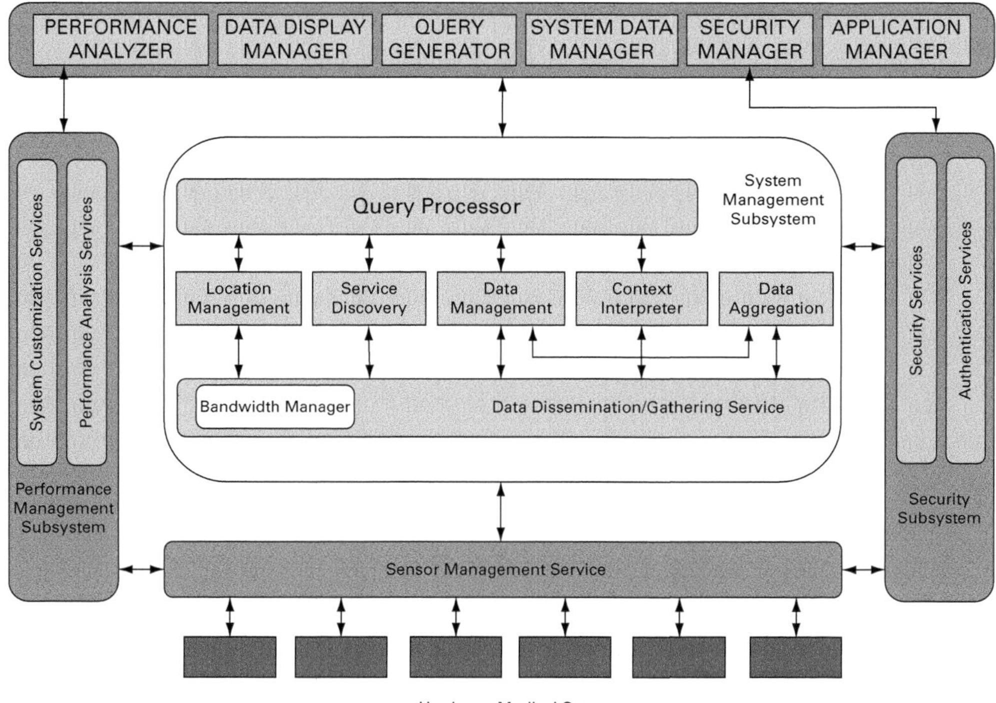

Figure 2.9   The architecture of a PHMS.

the Ayushman PHMS [53], shown in Figure 2.8, which was developed at the IMPACT Lab at the ASU. The Ayushman PHMS has five subcomponents: (1) context sensing, which senses environmental and physiological signals to facilitate the detection of user context; (2) context processing, which processes the sensed signals to determine the user context and perform necessary computations for the PHMS services; (3) data communication, which deals with the transfer of information from the sensors via the base station to the server; (4) energy sources, which determines the technology for energy supply to the sensors, base station, and server; and (5), last but not least, the human body with which the PHMS devices interact either through sensing and actuation or through harmful side-effects of operation such as thermal harm.

The typical architecture of the middleware for PHMSes is shown in Figure 2.9.

- At the lowest layer are the hardware medical sensors, which measure medical and other context information (location, time, physical state, work state) from patients. The information from the sensors is passed on to a sensor-management-services layer, which provides an abstraction of the hardware to the upper-layer services. The upper layer can control the working of the sensors through a standardized interface provided by the sensor-management-services layer.

- The sensor-management-services layer forwards the sensor data to a system-management subsystem, which provides services for effective patient health monitoring. Some of the services provided are listed below.

- Data-dissemination and -gathering service. This service provides effective communication primitives for gathering and disseminating data within the infrastructure, and it often uses multicasting, flooding, and unicast primitives. It also implements a bandwidth manager, which manages the allocation of bandwidth resources to various components of the infrastructure.
  - Location-management service. This is used to provide location information on patients, doctors, and equipment within a medical facility on the basis of sensor data.
  - Context-interpreter service. This is used to interpret a patient's context information sent by the sensors.
  - Data-management service. A PHMS is typically designed to collect both medical and administrative data from patients. In order to manage the data it collects, it provides two functions: buffer management and storage management. The former is used mostly for synchronization between different parts of the system after a recent disconnection, while the latter is used mostly for long-term storage of medical data.
  - Service-discovery service. A medical facility provides many services, and it is essential for an automated medical monitoring system to be able to discover them, register them, and present information about them when queried. A PHMS's service discovery allows applications to search for available medical services.
  - Data-aggregation service. A PHMS will collect lots of health-related data for each patient, and it is essential to be able to aggregate, analyze, and extract information from such data. The results of the data analysis and aggregated values are sent to the data-management service for appropriate storage.
  - Query-processing service. This service receives queries from the application layer, queries the above-mentioned services, and sends the data back. It can be used to query any information about the infrastructure, such as location, medical and administrative data, and context information.
- The middleware for BAN-based PHMSes is also designed to monitor and control the performance of the BAN hardware and software. In this regard, it provides a performance-management subsystem. The idea is to allow developers to plug in their protocols, change the properties of the system, and measure the protocol's performance. Two services enable this feature.
  - Performance-analysis service. This is a cross-layer service that is used to obtain performance metrics from the system-management service. This is different from the query processor, which queries patient-related data.
  - System-customization services. This is another cross-layer service, which, on a cue from an application, can change the properties of the system (e.g., change the bandwidth available to specific medical sensors). This can be used by protocol developers to test their work under different conditions.
- Medical information that a PHMS collects has to be kept secure in order to maintain patients' privacy. The Health Insurance Privacy and Accountability Act (HIPAA) laws [2] in the USA mandate that any electronic medical record has to be secure in order to prevent unauthorized access. Since security is important at all levels, a PHMS includes another cross-layer service for providing security and authentication

to all layers within the system through the security subsystem. The security subsystem can be controlled from the application layer to provide variable levels of security to different parts of the PHMS.

- The top-most layer of a PHMS is the application layer, which provides applications for managing the whole system. Some of the applications provided are listed below.
  - Performance analyzer. This interacts with the performance-management subsystem, and can be used by developers to monitor and control system properties.
  - Data display. This application is used for providing a meaningful way of displaying a patient's medical data.
  - Query generator. This is used to query data from the system, which it does by contacting the query processor.
  - System data manager. This is used to monitor and interpret all medical and administrative data in the system.
  - Security manager. This is used to monitor the system's security settings and to change them when needed.
  - Application manager. This application, as the name suggests, is used to monitor and manage resource allocation for all other applications.

2.4 Questions

1. Why are body area networks (BANs) designed to be wireless? What are the advantages or disadvantages of using wired communication channels with BANs?
2. Apart from wired and wireless communication between sensors, is there any other option (another path/conduit/channel) for communicating between sensors? If so, what are the advantages and disadvantages of using the option?
3. What are the different topologies in which a BAN can be organized? Discuss the pros and cons of each topology.
4. What are the hazards that operation of a BAN can cause to the human body?
5. Patient privacy is an essential part of securing BANs. What are the consequences of losing privacy with respect to medical/health data?
6. Identify the various sources of energy available from the human body to power sensors in a BAN. Compare them with respect to the energy they provide.
7. Analyze the solution proposed as part of Question 4 of Chapter 1. Discuss the potential safety, security, and sustainability of this solution, and suggest improvements.
8. Are cyber-physical systems different from the embedded systems which they replace? Why?

3   BAN models and requirements

In this book, we mainly focus on the pervasive health-monitoring system (PHMS), where the BAN nodes act as medical devices. Stand-alone BANs are typically ineffective due to their low computation and storage capability and limited battery life, especially when used in a PHMS setting. Thus, in PHMSes a BAN is usually used in conjunction with high-end embedded devices such as the smart phone and cloud-based computational and storage resources. Figure 3.1 shows the basic hardware architecture of a PHMS with the BAN deployed on the human body, communicating to a smart phone, which has limited storage and higher computation capability. The smart phone in turn uses the cloud for further processing and storage related to diagnosis and other applications. There have been different implementations of this basic architecture of a PHMS, each assuming different capabilities of the BAN, smart phone, and cloud. From a survey of the health-monitoring applications available on the market (at the time of writing this book), three categories of PHMS implementations have been identified.

- In the first category, the sensors are considered to be merely data-collection units with no computation and storage. The sensors are merely monitoring devices and are not approved as marketable medical devices by the FDA in the USA. The smart phone acts as the primary computation device; it performs signal processing on the physiological signals and displays results to the user. Most of these applications are not connected to the cloud or use the cloud as mere storage. Applications that fall within this category include the heart phone (`http://techcrunch.com/2011/05/24/smartheart-turns-your-mobile-phone-into-a-heart-monitor/`) and the ECG monitor app (`http://alivecor.com/`), which use sensors to obtain the physiological signals and the computation capability of the smart phone to show properties of the signals to the user.
- The second category of applications employs sensors as mere data-collection units, smart phones as data forwarders and display units, and the cloud as the main storage and computation unit. Such architectures are assumed by applications such as medical imaging using smart phones (`http://www.msnbc.msn.com/id/44761864/ns/technology_and_science-innovation/t/iphones-transform-medical-imaging-devices/`) and embryo-monitoring apps (`http://www.umm.edu/ency/article/003405.htm`).
- The third category of applications uses medical devices as sensors on the human body that are capable of decision making and actuation. Smart phones are used as controllers or display devices, while the cloud provides storage. Applications

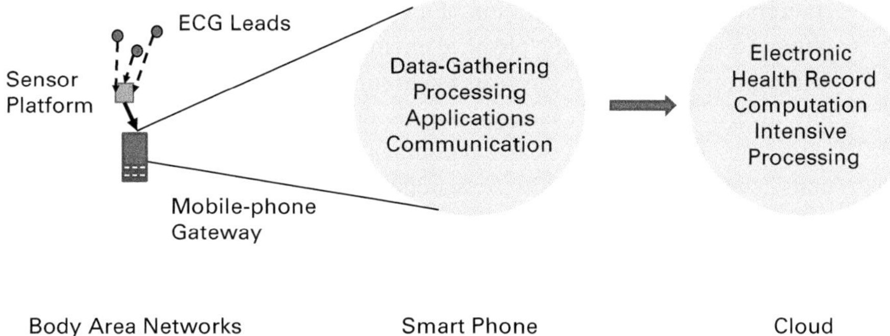

Figure 3.1 A body area network for pervasive health monitoring.

developed on these architectures are used in critical medical care facilities. Examples include network-controlled infusion pumps [50] and Holter monitors (`http://www.heartsite.com/html/holter.html`).

Irrespective of the extent to which BANs are used in the PHMS setting, they have to be designed in a manner that makes them effective and efficient. In this book, we consider the three principal requirements of BANs which enable this.

3.1 Principal requirements

The work in the domain of BANs thus far has principally focused on the infrastructural aspect of deploying BANs and collecting meaningful and error-free data. This has resulted in the development and availability of numerous BAN platforms. This book builds on these preliminary ideas and looks at BANs from a different perspective, namely their cyber-physical nature. This allows us to re-imagine the design of specific elements of BANs with respect to addressing the potential hazards due to their operation. In this regard, the book focuses on three aspects of BANs: (1) safety, namely ensuring that physical side-effects of operations remain within desired limits; (2) security, namely ensuring that only authorized actions on the system are performed; and (3) sustainability, namely ensuring uninterrupted operation of the BAN. In this section, we provide an overview of the principal issues associated with safety, security, and sustainability properties (collectively called S3 properties) in the context of BANs.

Before proceeding further, it should be noted that, although there are other issues in BAN design, such as reliability, data management, and real-time operation, in the context of this book we assume that these properties are subsumed into the overarching S3 issues. For example, if the communication link from an SpO_2 sensor in a BAN to the base station were unreliable, detection of cardiac emergencies would fail, endangering patient safety.

3.1.1 Safety

Safety is essential given the mission-critical deployments of BANs in health management. Standard ISO 60601 defines safety as the avoidance of hazards to the physical environment due to the operation of a medical device under normal or single-fault conditions [54]. Hazards in the physical environment can occur due to abnormal conditions in the properties of the physical environment, in this case the human body. Usually this involves creating a hazard-analysis document such as ISO 14971 that identifies harm caused to the physical environment due to faulty operation of the computing units (sensors). Traditionally, researchers have focused on bypassing this characterization and transforming the safety-assurance problem into a well-understood problem in computer science such as formal model-reachability analysis. In this regard, several static assumptions on the sensors/devices have been considered, which abstract out the dynamic nature of the physical environment. For example, in works such as [55, 56] infusion-pump software has been modeled using timed automata. The diffusion process is simplified so that the drug concentration in the blood is incremented by the infusion rate instantaneously. Such a simplified notion of safety, however, might not entirely capture the hazards resulting from the dynamic interactions of sensors/devices in BANs with their physical environment. Hence, in order to guarantee safety in BANs, it is necessary to accurately characterize the spatio-temporal dynamics of the physical environment and its tight coupling with the sensors/devices. Consequently, when dealing with the problem of safety assurance one needs to also consider interaction safety between the sensors and the physical environment, apart from the current focus on building bug-free software for sensors and medical devices.

Hazards due to lack of interaction safety can be of many different types.

- Interactions of two devices that are parts of different systems may affect each other's operation in hazardous ways. For example, headphones have been reported to interfere with pacemakers of heart patients (`http://www.medicaldevicesafety.org/`). The electromagnetic interaction of the headphone with the patient's body becomes coupled with the electromagnetism induced by the pacemaker on the patient's heart and deactivates it.
- Interaction between the sensors and the physical environment may have harmful effects on the physical environment, e.g., heating of skin/tissue surrounding a sensor due to its operation. Excessive electroporation and/or field effects may cause necrosis.
- The operation of the physical environment may hinder the operation of the sensors. For example, tissue growth around the implanted sensors can hamper sensing and communication capabilities.

Addressing the safety of interactions is a challenging task. Principally, it requires exact understanding of the physical processes of the environment and the properties of the computing unit which affect the physical processes.

3.1.2   Security

In the context of this book, we define security, rather generally, as the ability to ensure that both data and operational capabilities of the system, including sensing, communication, storage, processing, and actuation, can be accessed only when authorized. Security for BANs is a relatively new area. As with any new field, most of the effort seems to be focused on efficiently mapping solutions from existing domains [11]. The need for security in BANs is many-fold. Some of the main factors are listed below.

- *Mission-critical nature*. Their mandate for monitoring physiological parameters from the human body renders BANs mission-critical in nature. Therefore, any compromise of the sensors/devices and base station or the data communicated between them has profound consequences. A case in point is the attack on pacemakers which not only forced them to reveal a patient's electrocardiogram (ECG) data but also actuated untimely shocks [57].
- *Information sensitivity*. BANs collect a lot of sensitive health information about a person. If this information is available to malicious entities, it can be exploited, leading to loss of privacy, abuse, and discrimination. For example, unauthorized knowledge of the presence of a chronic condition of a person can lead to advertent/inadvertent bias from potential employers or insurers.
- *Ability to actuate*. The ability to actuate changes to the patient's body is increasingly being delegated to BANs. Allowing unauthorized parties to actuate untimely changes can cause harm to the patient. For example, malicious entities can easily shut down the automated infusion of insulin after a meal, causing a dangerous increase in blood glucose levels.
- *Ubiquity*. As BANs become viable and their presence becomes common, the incentive for attacking them for profit goes up. Consequently, it is essential to think about security in advance and have mature security solutions ready for them before they are deployed *en masse*.

Addressing security in BANs presents numerous challenges. First, the deployment of BANs is not limited to specialized systems managed by tech-savvy people. Many of the deployments of BAN systems will be for everyday use, in which they will be operated by non-technical people. Therefore, security solutions for BANs should have a high degree of *usability*, a characteristic that today's security solutions only minimally possess. Further, BANs are made up of devices and sensors that are heterogeneous and have limited capabilities. Therefore, security solutions for BANs need to be effective and *lightweight* enough to be executable on platforms available as part of BANs. Further, they have to be *flexible* enough to be able to adapt to the different operational situation of BANs, ranging from normal situations to emergencies.

Our approach to achieving these is through the use of information from the physical environment. This enables us to meet the security needs of BANs while satisfying the challenges presented above.

3.1.3　Sustainability

Sustainability from a BAN standpoint can be defined as the balance between the power required by the sensors for computation and the power available from various energy sources. Traditionally, sensors in BANs have been supplied energy from the battery. However, with the recent push towards alternative green sources of energy the energy-supply model has changed. There are two possible energy-supply models: (1) where the harvesting/scavenging source directly supplies energy to the computing unit, the scavenging-source-to-computing-system (SSCS) model; and (2) where the scavenging source first stores the energy to a battery and then the battery supplies energy to the computing unit, the scavenging-source-to-battery-to-computing-system (SBCS) model. The energy-supply model imposes several challenges on the sustainable design of BANs.

- *Intermittent energy supply.* Environmental energy sources are inherently intermittent in nature. Hence there is no guarantee that the power needs of the BAN will be met at every time instant. For the SSCS model, often the power supply and demand do not match. For the SBCS model there is energy wastage when the amount of power obtained is greater than the amount the battery can store. To achieve a sustainable BAN design, the power demand from the sensors has to be matched by the power scavenged from various sources at all time instants, while at the same time minimizing waste.
- *Unknown load characteristics.* The operating voltage obtained across the sensors depends on the input impedance and the load characteristics of the source. For green energy sources the voltage and current are often related through a convex function [58]. The power drawn from the source is maximum at a certain voltage and current. Hence for maximum efficiency the optimal operating voltage and current have to be determined from the load characteristic.

The properties of the physical environment, which are utilized to scavenge energy, such as the intensity of sunlight, and the body temperature, affect the amount of energy available to power computing units. The computing properties, such as the allowable duty cycle, frequency of operation, and server utilization, need to be adjusted on the basis of the available energy in order to make the overall BAN design more sustainable.

3.2   The cyber-physical nature of BANs

Before we delve into the details of designing BANs to satisfy the S3 properties, it is essential to give an overview of our unique perspective in addressing them, taking into account the *cyber-physical* nature of the BAN operation, which is based on the interaction of the sensors with their environment (the human body).

As mentioned in the previous section, a major characteristic of BANs is their tight coupling with the physical environment. The term used to describe such systems is *cyber-physical* systems. A cyber-physical system (CPS) consists of embedded computing units, which frequently interact with their physical environment to provide important functionalities. In the case of a BAN, this involves monitoring a patient's health and actuating treatment if necessary. The *computing units* of a CPS can be characterized by a set of properties. These properties are related to the computing operation and are functions of the application being executed by the computation unit. The *physical environment* in a CPS can be similarly characterized by a set of quantitative properties, for example physiological and environmental signals such as the level of blood glucose, temperature, and humidity.

In a CPS, the computing properties closely interact with physical properties through a *physical process*. The process, depending upon the operation of the computing units, can cause variations in the physical environment and vice versa. Typical examples of such processes include the infusion of drugs, heat dissipation through the tissue due to the operation of the sensor, and complex features extracted from physiological signals. The first two are examples of the computing unit using the process to affect the process, while the last one is an example of the process affecting the computing unit's operation.

The properties of the physical environment vary over both space and time. For example, the temperature of the body varies at different locations within the body. As cyber-physical systems, BANs exhibit spatio-temporal dynamics.

Example 3.1. Consider a BAN with a fingertip pulse-oximeter operation. The sampling frequency of the oximeter affects the amount of heat dissipated into the surrounding tissue. The effect of the dissipated heat on the rise of the tissue temperature is characterized by the Pennes bioheat equation [59]. Such a mapping is an example of spatio-temporal dynamics.

In general, cyber-physical interactions can be of two types: (1) *intended interactions*, namely the usage of information from the physical environment for performing useful computing operations; and (2) *unintended interactions*, namely the side-effects of operation of the computing units on the physical environment. Further, in the case of networked CPSes, there are often combined effects of the individual interactions, called *aggregate effects*, as observed in multi-channel drug infusion. A case in point is the increased death rate of cancerous cells when a monoclonal antibody and methotrexate drugs are infused simultaneously in comparison with when they are infused sequentially [60].

We can categorize the work-flow of a typical CPS into three main functions. (1) *Monitoring*. The most fundamental aspect of a CPS deals with monitoring the physical process within the CPS. It is also used to provide feedback on any past actions taken by the CPS and to ensure correct operations in the future. (2) *Processing*. This deals with analyzing the data collected during monitoring to determine whether the physical process is meeting certain pre-defined criteria. In situations where the criteria are not being satisfied, corrective actions are determined, which, when executed, ensure that the criteria are satisfied. For example, a data-center CPS can observe its thermal characteristics, and then develop a model to predict the temperature rise with respect to various scheduling algorithms, which can be used to determine future jobs [61]. (3) *Actuation*. This deals with executing the actions determined during the data-processing phase. Actuation can take many forms, from changing the behavior of the cyber element to changing the physical process itself, for example, delivery of medicine and authorizing access to data collected by a BAN. This work-flow of a CPS can execute in one of three possible modes (see Figure 3.2).

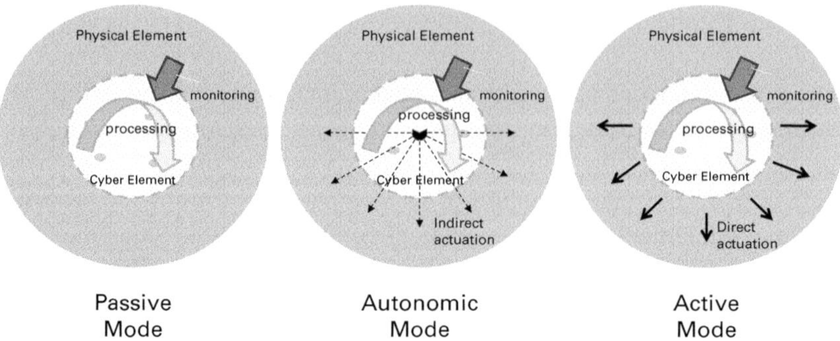

Figure 3.2   Operational modes of cyber-physical systems.

- *Passive.* In this mode, CPSes act as information-gathering platforms only, and solely monitor their constituent physical processes, processing the data, e.g., medical devices such as pulse oximeters.
- *Autonomic.* In this mode, CPSes monitor their constituent physical processes and, if they see some property not being satisfied, they execute an indirect actuation by changing their own behavior (the cyber aspect) so that the property can be satisfied, for example, data centers performing smart scheduling to minimize temperature rises at specific spots.
- *Active.* In this mode, CPSes monitor their constituent physical processes and, if some property is not being satisfied, they execute a direct actuation by modifying the behavior of the process to ensure that the property is satisfied, for example, an HVAC (heating, ventilating, and air conditioning) unit in a building blowing cold air into the building if the temperature exceeds a certain established limit.

Not all CPSes need implement all these modes of operation. Some may implement one or a particular combination of modes. The BANs we consider in this book usually are assumed to operate in the passive category. However, this does not mean that the solutions proposed do not apply when the BAN is operated in the other two modes. Many issues need to be addressed in order to make each of these types of CPS system viable, such as managing the cyber and physical interactions, and ensuring safety, energy efficiency, interoperability, and sustainability. Indeed, it is this perspective that allows us to tackle the S3 issues, which form the core of this book, in a manner that has not been considered before, utilizing information from and about the physical environment in order to design BANs such that they are safe, secure, and can achieve sustained operation.

Apart from the S3 issues BANs are also regulated by the government for safety. A BAN designer has to follow these regulations in order to market the manufactured devices. In the following section, we go through the regulatory issues that different government agencies impose on BAN designers.

3.3 Regulatory issues

Given the sensitive and safety-critical nature of medical devices, the firms that produce such devices are regulated by a governmental authority. Throughout the world medical-device regulatory bodies exist. In the USA, the Food and Drug Administration (FDA) is the federal agency with the remit for this task. More specifically, the Center for Devices and Radiological Health (CDRH) within the FDA is responsible for regulating firms that manufacture, repackage, relabel, and/or import medical devices and radiation-emitting products sold within the USA [62]. In the EU, the manufacturers of medical devices are required to obtain certification from the European Committee for Standardization (CEN) and the European Committee for Electrotechnical Standardization (Cenelec). In Asia, different countries have their own medical-device regulatory agencies through which the certification process is handled. A recent survey by Pacific Bridge Medical (`http://www.pacificbridgemedical.com/`) lists China and India as the leading medical-device users in Asia. In China, the regulatory agency is the State Food and Drug Administration (SFDA), while in India it is the Central Drugs Standard Control Organisation (CDSCO). In the following sections we will discuss some of the salient features of the regulatory strategies in the USA, the EU, and Asia.

3.3.1 Medical-device regulation in the USA

The FDA classifies medical devices into three categories: classes I, II, and III. *Class I* devices are usually minimally scrutinized, and their manufacturers are exempt from providing any notification. *Class II* devices usually require Pre-market Notification 510(k), which essentially states that the marketed medical device is substantially equivalent to existing cleared medical devices or a device in use before 1976. Most *class III* devices require pre-market approval. Such devices usually pose significant risk of injury or are so new that there are no other devices on the market to which substantial equivalence can be proven. Manufacturers of devices classified as class III have to provide substantial clinical data to support their case.

Thus far safety has been the fundamental goal of medical-device manufacturers and the FDA in the past. This has led to the development of a process for ensuring safety properties using tools such as (1) *failure modes and effects analysis (FMEA) (JC14.3)* and (2) *hazard analysis (ISO 14971)*. Manufacturers must convince the FDA that they have accounted for and mitigated all safety hazards. Recently, safety in the context of security has become a growing issue. As healthcare technology evolves to include more sophisticated communication interfaces, with device interoperability on the horizon, federal regulators such as the FDA face new challenges.

Several approaches to enable medical-device security are being considered. For instance, manufacturers may need to provide the user with appropriate device-interface information and information to adequately configure communication systems with regard to managing security issues. Further, it could be the user's responsibility to address physical security issues, such as tampering with a device. The FDA has issued a cyber-security guidance document that addresses some of the security issues (Cybersecurity for networked medical devices containing off the shelf (OTS) software, available from `http://www.fda.gov/cdrh/comp/guidance/1553.html`). Work is also being done to look at security from a medical-device safety and risk-management perspective. The draft International Electrotechnical Commission (IEC) 80001 standard (`http://www.iec.ch`) on risk management includes security considerations, but again from a security administration and software-design perspective.

At the time of writing, security in medical devices has started to be addressed. The FDA is working on a guidance document to make device manufacturers explicitly address security concerns in their 510(k) submissions to the FDA. In particular, the manufacturers are expected to describe how their software addresses information-security issues, especially its four main aspects: *confidentiality* (data and information about data and its generation are accessible only to authorized personnel), *integrity* (data generated are complete and have not been modified in an unauthorized manner), *availability* (data and service are available, in a timely manner, as required), and *accountability* (an authorized user is identified and authenticated before use). Further, if the device has a wireless interface then detailed information needs to be given about the data which will be transmitted wirelessly, quality of service needed, security protocols used, and potential interference from other radiofrequency (RF) technologies. For devices that store and display data, in general medical-device data systems (MDDSes) should undertake measures for preserving data privacy.

In addition, the FDA will also require manufacturers to provide assurance cases for characterizing the safety and security features of the medical device. *Assurance cases* represent a framework for arguing that evidence justifies a claim. They provide a means for convincing a third party, such as a regulator, that a particular claim is justified. For medical-device security, one might claim that the device is adequately secure for its intended use in a particular use environment. Developing assurance cases like their safety counterpart is a three-step process, involving *claims*, *arguments*, and *evidence*, as follows. (1) Specifying the claims about certain properties of the system, for example, that communication between devices and the network controller is secure. (2) Making arguments about the evidence justifying the claim, for example, the use of an encryption algorithm for hiding (i.e., encrypting) data communicated between the device and the network controller. (3) Providing evidence to support the arguments made regarding the claim, for example, AES algorithm implementation is verified via formal proof documentation or reasoned test cases that are verified via documentation. Building assurance cases for individual components of the medical device system is not sufficient. Eventually, the individual assurance cases have to be composed as well, to satisfy security claims regarding the entire system. Finally, developing assurance cases also involves providing cost–benefit justification for their use [63].

A recent report by the Institute of Medicine at the National Academy of Sciences, Medical Devices and the Public's Health: The FDA's 510(k) Clearance Process at 35 Years, however, has cast doubt on this entire process of clearing high-risk medical devices and has recommended a complete overhaul of the clearance process. In this regard, the 510(k) process of substantial equivalence has come under question since two-thirds of all high-risk devices recalled since 2005 had been cleared in this manner. The 510(k) rule was set in place to expedite the clearance of medical devices, thereby increasing the rate at which new devices became available to patients. However, expediting the introduction into use of new devices without the requirement of detailed clinical data (unlike pharmaceutical drugs) solely on the basis of an imprecisely described notion of substantial equivalence has become problematic.

3.3.2　Medical-device regulation in the EU

Medical device certification in Europe follows a different procedure than that employed by the FDA in the USA. The certification procedure first classifies medical devices into two classes: minimal risk and greater risk. This distinction is done according to certain *directives* published by the CEN. For the minimal-risk devices, a self-certification procedure is followed. Here the manufacturers prepare a *declaration-of-conformity* document claiming their device to be of minimal risk and themselves put the CE mark on the device. For the greater-risk devices, the certification directives require them to be independently certified. This independent certification must be done by a *notified body*, which is an organization that is nominated by the government and has been notified by the European Commission. The notified bodies serve as independent labs and perform the steps listed in the directives to check conformity of the device and process. Manufacturers may choose a notified body in any member state of the European Union. Lists of notified bodies are published by the European Commission in the Official Journal of the European Union.

3.3.3　Medical-device regulation in Asia

In Asia, each country has its own regulatory body to standardize medical devices. The primary users of medical devices, China and India, import considerable amounts of devices from the USA and the EU. In this context, authorizing agencies such as the FDA and the CEN are recognized in China and India, and no further regulation is performed.

In India specifically, about 75% of the medical devices are imports that have already been pre-verified. However, recently the government has issued a list of 10 medical devices including cardiac and drug-eluting stents that require central clearance prior to marketing. A National Drug Authority has been set up, which, apart from monitoring drugs and clinical trials, will also evaluate the safety of the medical devices. On the other hand, in China, the SFDA has taken a series of steps to quicken the process of medical-device certification. For low-risk medical devices the certification procedure can take as little as 15 minutes.

4   Safety

This chapter focuses on the various definitions, challenges, and approaches to BAN safety. Standard ISO 60601, a standard for medical devices, defines safety as the avoidance of unacceptable risks of hazards to the physical environment (i.e., to the patient) due to the operation of a medical device under normal or single-fault condition. Although this definition is akin to that for medical devices, it can be generally applicable to BANs as well, which are essentially networks of such devices. The standard further lists seven aspects of safety as follows.

1. *Operational aspect.* This aspect considers safety as the correct (and error-free) operation of the medical device, which might involve software, hardware, and electrical and mechanical operations, as well as the usage of medical devices in clinical processes (or medical scenarios).
2. *Radiation aspect.* This aspect of safety is geared towards ensuring that any radiation (e.g., X-ray radiation) from the device does not harm the patient.
3. *Thermal aspect.* This aspect of safety concerns the need to ensure that any heat dissipated because of medical-device operation and power consumption does not burn any part of the patient's body.
4. *Biocompatibility.* This aspect requires the materials used for the medical device to be compatible with the human body.
5. *Software aspect.* This aspect is essentially covered under the operational aspect; however, with the proliferation of software-enabled devices and sensors, special emphasis has been placed on correct operation of device software (e.g., code consistency and execution flow).
6. *Mechanical aspect.* This aspect principally requires that any actuation (e.g., the infusion process employed by an infusion pump) from the medical device does not cause harm to the body.
7. *Electrical aspect.* This aspect is intended to ensure that the device does not deliver any electrical shock to the body.

Note that the basic objective of all the safety aspects is to avoid harm being caused to patients by medical devices. Although the manifestation of this objective (and potential harm to the patient) may be different for different safety aspects, it is important to understand that safety of a BAN essentially means safety of the patient on whom the BAN is deployed. The principal question therefore is, given all the different aspects, that of how to ensure *patient safety*.

4.1   Safety approaches

In this section, we elaborate on various approaches to BAN safety. We first provide a perspective on BAN safety taking into consideration its usage model, its network-centric focus, and the increasing reliance on software.

4.1.1   Perspectives of BAN safety

Traditionally, safety engineers have focused on bypassing the characterization of patient safety and transforming the patienty-safety-assurance problem into a well-understood problem in computer science. In this regard, principally, there are three different safety perspectives.

Scenario safety

From the perspective of the medical scenario and clinical processes the main idea behind safety is to develop methodologies to handle critical physiological conditions in the hospital. It is important that for a series of critical events the correct methodologies are followed to mitigate all of them. Example research in this regard includes the criticality-response planning, evaluation, and actuation [64, 65].

Example 4.1. Consider a hospital with bed-ridden patients, an intensive-care unit (ICU), and outpatient facilities. Plans are established to handle several critical scenarios, such as an influx of emergency patients, an excess of outpatients during pandemics, and critical ICU patients. However, many other criticalities, such as fire hazards and earthquakes, can occur in a hospital. Scenario safety deals with ensuring that the strategies employed to mitigate such criticalities are truly effective. Also, in the case of multiple criticalities occurring simultaneously a scenario-safety analysis will ensure that a mitigative action does not introduce other criticalities and that after a sequence of mitigative actions the system reaches a state in which all criticalities are mitigated.

Network safety

Many medical responses would involve a network of medical devices, so it is important to analyze the impact of network delays and packet drops on critical-care operations. Such an evaluation of patient safety in medical-device networks has been performed by Gehlot *et al.* of Villanova University [66]. Further, human mobility causes changes in the wireless environment of the medical devices in the BAN. Such changes due to mobility can cause packet drops, which may in turn result in safety hazards. Network-safety analysis under human mobility has been considered by Banerjee and Gupta [67]. The authors conclude that safe configurations of medical devices can have hazardous operations for certain mobility patterns. Specifically, simulations of a network-controlled infusion pump show that user mobility can change the properties of the communication medium, causing loss of control commands, which may lead to drug-overdose hazards.

Example 4.2. Consider an ECG-monitoring device such as a Holter monitor being controlled by a server through the wireless channel. The wireless channel is prone to errors that cause loss of control information. This may cause abnormal conditions such as arrhythmia to remain unnoticed.

Example 4.3. Consider a network of low-power sensor devices, e.g., ECG sensors, interfaced with the TelosB motes. A cluster-based multi-hop communication protocol is used [68] for the network. In this protocol, the sensor nodes in the BAN form a cluster. Nodes in a cluster nominate a leader node, a.k.a. the cluster head. All the non-leader nodes transmit their sensed data to the cluster head. The cluster head then forwards these data to the base station, and hence has a pretty high communication workload. The absorption of electromagnetic radiation (because of communication) can cause heat dissipation, which in turn may lead to significant thermal effects in the surrounding human tissue [69].

Software safety

Software safety is directly related to the behavior of the software in the system. An example of software-safety analysis is verification of whether an infusion pump issues an alarm on detecting an abnormal increase in the infusion rate [49]. There are three different aspects of software safety.

1. *Code safety*, which concerns safety from coding errors such as infinite while loops, unreachable conditions etc. as performed in the Generic Infusion Pump project at the University of Pennsylvania [49].
2. *Control-system safety*, which concerns safety from undershoot, overshoot, instability, and long settling times (investigated as part of the model-predictive control system design of infusion pumps [70]).
3. *Interaction safety*, which concerns the interactions of a medical-device control system with the human physiology [71]. Medical devices, such as infusion pumps, often receive feedback from the human body or actuate critical medical operations such as drug infusion to control the physiology. The operation of the software is governed by the changes in the human physiology. Interaction safety ensures that the medical device does not cause harm to the user given the continuous interaction.

Example 4.4. Consider a fingertip pulse oximeter used for monitoring the heart rate of an infant. Obtaining each sample for a pulse oximeter requires passage of light through the fingertip tissue. The passage of light causes heat transfer to the fingertip. A high sampling rate may cause excessive heat transfer to the fingertip skin and hence may result in burn hazards. This phenomenon has been noted in several clinical studies [72].

Example 4.5. Consider an infusion pump, being controlled by a smart phone, which can be used for infusion of either insulin or analgesic. Further, the controller algorithm uses feedback from a pulse oximeter or glucose sensor and computes the drug-infusion rate to control the blood glucose level or the level of consciousness. The infusion-pump software can have bugs such as infinite loops and memory overflows. The controller may receive faulty values from the sensors. Moreover, the communication between the sensor and the smart phone might break, leading to lack of feedback. The effect of these errors can lead to a fatal drug overdose and possible physiological hazards such as respiratory distress [50] and low blood sugar level.

The Food and Drug Administration (FDA) has been actively involved in ensuring software safety of medical devices.

4.1.2 Ensuring BAN safety

There are four different approaches in this regard.

The experimental approach

In this approach, specific experiments are performed to characterize the effects of the medical device on human physiology. An example of where such an approach is used is thermal safety evaluation of a pulse oximeter [73]. However, such an approach can be applicable for other types of safety evaluation, provided that appropriate experiments can be designed and that the risk to human and/or animal subjects has been mitigated appropriately.

The emulation approach

In this approach, hardware models for human body parts are developed, and devices are tested on the hardware models. Examples of such an approach include using heart models to extensively test the operation of pacemakers [74]. This approach can be used mostly for device software and control-system safety evaluation.

Software testing

This approach involves simulation of the medical device on a huge set of test cases, e.g., infusion-pump software testing [49]. This approach can be used for testing device software code and networks.

Software verification

This approach uses formal models to characterize the device behavior and analysis methodology for these models to provide safety guarantees. For example, timed automata have been used to model the behavior of an infusion pump [75]. This approach can be applicable to evaluate the safety of software code, a network, a control system, and a medical scenario.

The last two approaches fall within the much more generic methodology of software engineering.

All of these approaches suffer either from static abstractions of the human body or from the infeasibility of designing experimental scenarios (since actual deployments can be hazardous, intrusive, costly, and disastrous in the case of faulty or unsafe BAN operations). A more cyber-physically oriented automated approach that can abstract the cooperation of discrete-time software behavior and dynamic physical behavior (of the environment) is required. Such an abstraction should also represent the real deployment scenarios. The consequences of the BAN behavior on human physiology can then be analyzed to evaluate patient safety.

4.2   Model-based engineering of BANs

One method by which to evaluate safety is model-based engineering (MBE), which is the method of developing models of real systems and analyzing the models for requirement verification. Figure 4.1 depicts the different phases in this methodology. There are two main phases in MBE: (1) model development and (2) model analysis. In the model-development phase, a set of expected properties of the system is determined from the system requirements. An abstract modeling is further performed, which generally involves (i) capturing various components and their interactions that reflect the architecture of the systems or (ii) capturing appropriate parameters whose variations can reflect the system behavior. Analysis is then performed on the abstract model to evaluate the expected properties and verify the system requirements.

Several methodologies for safety-requirements analysis, high-level modeling of medical devices and BANs, and analysis of safety exist.

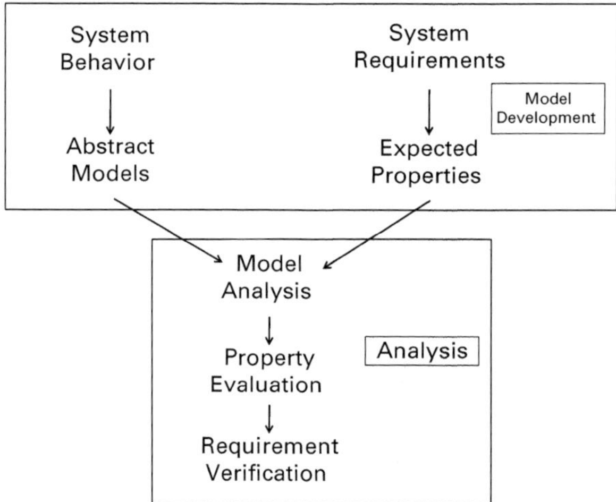

Figure 4.1   Model-based engineering methodology.

4.2.1   Safety-requirements analysis

Safety-requirements analysis begins with a hazard analysis of the medical device or BAN as recommended by the FDA [55]. In a hazard analysis, a medical device is first decomposed into subcomponents and connections between them [55]. For each subcomponent, possible failure modes are considered. These failure modes are obtained from the failure history of the medical device or careful evaluation of the system. Research at the FDA [55] has established a Simulink-based model of hazards for an infusion pump. The Simulink-based framework can generate random hazards and simulate the effect of the hazard on the infusion pump. These requirements are then put into a standard document, which is used as a reference by the manufacturer as hazard recommendations from the FDA. Ideas from security-requirements analysis can be applied in analyzing safety. Often swimlane diagrams are used to analyze the security requirements of a system. One considers a model of the attacker and the possible forms of attack that can occur. These are then translated into possible security vulnerabilities in the system. Each vulnerability is then mapped to the components of the system that can be improved to prevent the security attack. The concept of swimlane diagrams can be used to analyze the different safety requirements in a BAN. Figure 4.2 shows the swimlane diagram for the safety of an infusion pump, which is controlled over the network by a central controller.

As can be seen in Figure 4.2, there are three kinds of safety hazards considered, namely those pertaining to human control (excessive infusion), computer control (overshoot), and the pump mechanics (occlusion). For each type of hazard there are measures to mitigate the hazard. Thus a swimlane diagram can be used to identify the causes of possible safety vulnerabilities in the BAN.

4.2.2   Model generation

There are many tools available that model and analyze the hardware of computing systems, such as Pspice [76] and Architecture Analysis and Design Language (AADL)

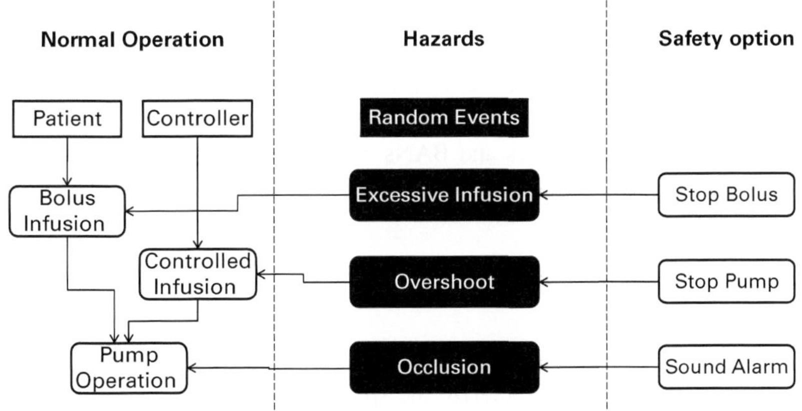

Figure 4.2   A swimlane diagram to analyze the safety requirements of an infusion pump.

(http://www.aadl.info/), and application software such as UML (http://www.uml.org/) and Petrinets [77]. Prasad *et al.* [78] have proposed a tool called ANDES that introduces the concept of MBE in WSNs to ensure accuracy and low latency of WSN operations. The MBE approach has also been used to study the behavior of physical systems through tools such as SysML (http://www.sysml.org/), Simulink (http://www.mathworks.com/), and Flovent (http://www.mentor.com/). A generic framework to perform MBE of CPSes has been proposed in [78]. However, the framework considers only the intentional interactions for the proper functioning of the CPSes. The MBE of BANs further needs to consider the un-intentional interactions in order to analyze BANs' safety. This chapter will present the BAND-AiDe tool, which provides a uniform model-specification and analysis platform that addresses the aforementioned modeling requirements for MBE of BANs.

Another branch of modeling is formal modeling, whereby operation of the medical device is represented as a collection of states and transitions between them. Such formal modeling has been undertaken by researchers [75] and several timed-automata, finite-state-machine (FSM)-based models have been proposed. Further, given the cyber-physical nature of the medical devices, several hazards, such as thermal radiation, might not be accurately analyzed using the FSM and timed automata. Hence, the use of spatio-temporal hybrid automata has been proposed in the literature [71] in order to capture such complex effects.

4.2.3   Analysis of safety

Given the two different types of modeling – architectural and formal – there can be two types of analysis performed on these models – simulation analysis and reachability analysis. Simulation analysis of safety on behavioral models has been considered by several researchers, using tools such as MATLAB®, Simulink®, and AADL. Reachability analysis for ensuring safety guarantees has been researched in the literature [79], and several theoretical methodologies have been proposed. However, these analysis techniques become overly complex when accurate models are used. Hence, simplifications of the models are performed, including linearization of models and the use of static assumptions on the dynamic parameters.

In the following sections, we will explore the difficulties in modeling BANs and the requirements in order for a safety-analysis technique to successfully guarantee safe operation of medical devices and BANs. We will then consider an example of a BAN safety-analysis tool that satisfies all the requirements set forth.

4.3   Modeling cyber-physical systems

Any model-based technique for ensuring the safety of cyber-physical systems, such as BANs, will need to characterize the spatio-temporal cyber-physical interactions (as described in Chapter 2). In this regard, Banerjee *et al.* [80] have proposed an abstract modeling framework for CPSes (GCPS) as shown in Figure 4.3.

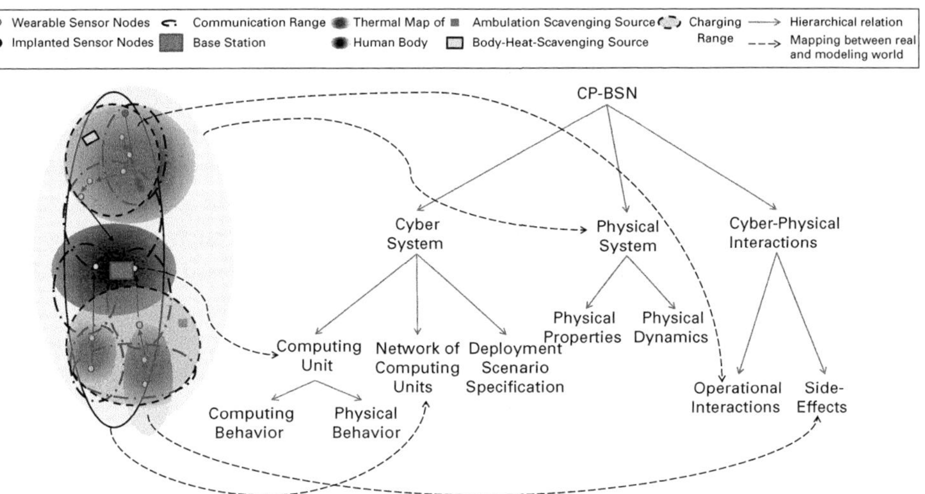

Figure 4.3   The BAN modeling requirements.

The CPS is considered as a network of several local CPSes (LCPSes). Each LCPS consists of a computing unit, interaction parameters, and two associated spatial regions of the physical environment: (a) the region of impact (ROIm) and (b) the region of interest (ROIn). Associated with each computing unit are computing properties (**C**), such as the frequency of operation, and physical properties of the computing unit (**P**), such as specific heat and temperature rise. The interaction parameters are common to the computing and the physical unit, and include parameters such as the heat transferred, air-flow rate, and infusion rate. The ROIn and ROIm characterize the spatial extents of the effects of the intended and unintended interactions, respectively. The ROIn or ROIm of an LCPS has three components.

- The *monitored parameter*, which is a property of the physical environment (**P**) and manifests the effects of the cyber-physical interactions. Typical examples include temperature, drug concentration, and cell-death rate.
- The *region boundary*, which signifies the spatial extent of the effect of interactions. The variation of the monitored parameters beyond this region is negligible.
- The *physical dynamics*, a model of the physical process governing the spatio-temporal variation of the monitored parameters. For example, it can be a multi-dimensional partial differential equation governing the temperature rise on the human body, namely Pennes' equation [59].

The GCPS model is the basic architectural model of any CPS and clearly incorporates the unified approach to CPS design by provisioning the constructs to model both the computing and the physical environment in the same framework. The GCPS models can be used for two purposes: (a) to check the consistency of models of CPS developed using specialized tools such as Ptolemy (`http://ptolemy.eecs.berkeley.edu/`) in specific domains and (b) to perform simulation analysis of any CPS. Since the GCPS model is generic and provides a comprehensive set of modeling constructs, it is a good candidate for the base architecture. Since systems from various domains are CPSes, specific modeling needs may give rise to specialized modeling tools. An important research problem in this regard is to check the consistency and the ability to capture cyber-physical inter-dependences of the models developed in different domains [81]. Recent research endeavors [81] have resulted in a typed-graph-based technique to show isomorphisms between different models of a CPS. In such a technique, the equivalence of different models to a base architecture is considered as a consistency check. The GCPS is a good candidate for the base architecture.

Given the model of a CPS, traditionally there are two methods to analyze it: (a) simulation analysis on a given set of test cases and (b) model checking, where the CPS model is represented using a formal method and theoretical guarantees on system properties are provided. In this chapter, BANs, which are examples of CPSes, are considered in order to show the use of CPS models both in simulation analysis and in model checking for safety.

4.4   Example: BAND-AiDe – BAN Design and Analysis Tool

This section presents the BAND-AiDe tool. Figure 4.4 shows the architecture of the tool and depicts how it enables the execution of the different phases in MBE. As shown in Figure 4.4, BAND-AiDe consists of a model-development framework, called the *BAND-AiDe modeling framework* (Section 4.4.1), and a model-analysis engine, called the *BAND-AiDe model analyzer* (Section 4.4.2).

4.4.1   The BAND-AiDe modeling framework

The modeling framework helps in the model-development phase of MBE (Figure 4.1). There are three inputs to the framework.

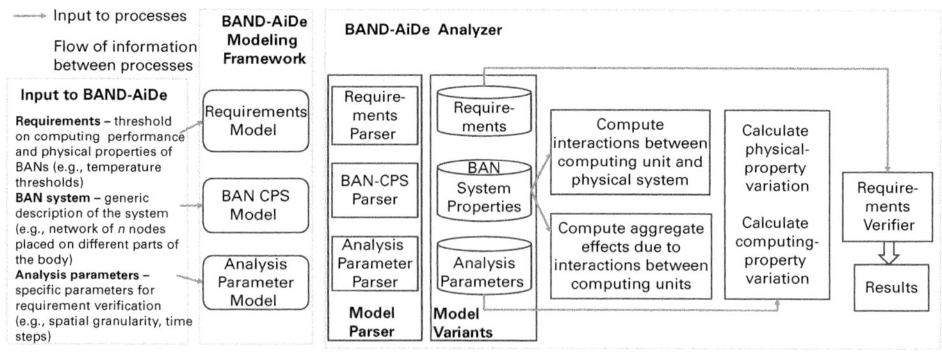

Figure 4.4   The BAND-AiDe tool architecture.

1. **BAN requirements**. These are usually a set of limits or thresholds on the system parameters. For example, an upper limit on the maximum body temperature (system parameter) ensures safety. Similarly, for BAN sustainability, the requirements are to ensure that at least a given number of nodes (system parameter) can be operated using available power from different energy resources.
2. **BAN system**. This includes BAN deployment information such as the number, types, spatial distribution, and communication topology of the nodes.
3. **Analysis parameters**. These are specific parameters for the model analysis. Examples of such parameters include time steps, the spatial granularity of differential-equation solvers (e.g., finite-difference time domain (FDTD) [69]), and functions determining the aggregate effects (e.g., a summation function to combine heat effects from multiple computing units).

Given these inputs, the following subsections describe modeling methodologies in the BAND-AiDe modeling framework.

Requirements modeling

The thresholds on the system parameters, which characterize the BAN requirements, can be modeled in BAND-AiDe by providing a set of **constants**. These constants will be used in the requirements-verification phase to check whether the BAN behavior is suitably constrained.

Abstract modeling of BANs as CPSes (BAN-CPS)

This modeling methodology is used on the **BAN system** inputs to model BAN behavior. BAND-AiDe envisions a BAN as a CPS, which consists of a set of computing (i.e., cyber) components (medical devices) and a physical environment (the human body). Figure 4.5 shows a typical deployment of the BAN nodes including both implanted and wearable (i.e., on the skin) sensor nodes. Both the intentional and the un-intentional interactions are further depicted in Figure 4.5. This CPS view of a BAN is termed a BAN-CPS. Figure 4.6 shows all the modeling constructs of BAN-CPS in a hierarchical form. The following are the modeling constructs.

Global CPS (GCPS). A BAN is considered as a GCPS (Figure 4.5), i.e., a collection of distributed and networked cyber-physical subsystems. Each of these subsystems consists of a single worker node. The GCPS construct can also correspond to the portion of the physical environment observed for analysis, e.g., the portion of the human body monitored by BANs.

Local CPS (LCPS). Each individual subsystem in a GCPS is referred to as an LCPS. The LCPS construct models each worker node in a BAN as a single CPS. This enables modeling and analysis of the interactions between each individual node and the physical environment in a modular fashion. Each LCPS consists of three types of constructs.

- The *computing unit*. This construct corresponds to the sensor nodes capable of sensing, computation, and communication. The construct facilitates the modeling of both computing and physical behavior of the sensor nodes through the following two properties.

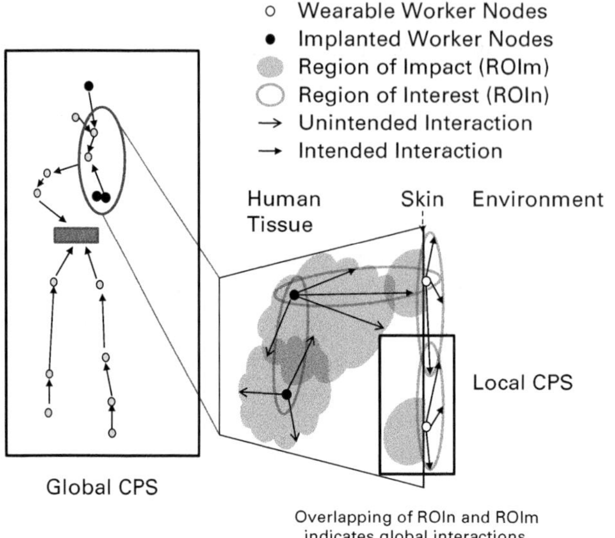

Figure 4.5   BAN-CPS: a BAN as a global cyber-physical system (CPS).

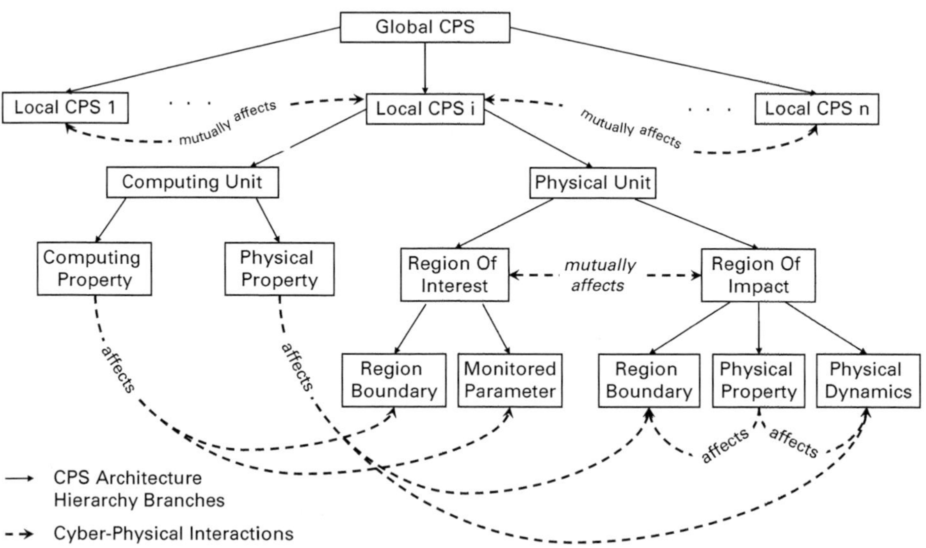

Figure 4.6   A hierarchical view of the generic constructs used to model BAN-CPS.

- The *computing property*. This property characterizes the computing behavior, e.g., the processor speed of a worker node or the amount of memory space available. The computing properties depend on the hardware configuration of the computing unit and the design of the application software. The hardware and the application software should be designed such that BAN operations are accurate and have low latency. These design requirements have been addressed in [82] and are beyond the scope of this chapter. Trade-offs of these design requirements with safety and sustainability are demonstrated in the specific case studies (Section 4.5).

– The *physical property*. This property characterizes the physical behavior, e.g., the power dissipation, of the computing unit. These properties often depend on the computing behavior of the nodes and can cause un-intentional interactions. For example, the processor speed determines the power dissipation of the sensor nodes. This in turn causes an un-intentional temperature rise of the human body.

- The *physical unit*. This construct is used to model the portion of the physical environment with which the computing unit interacts. These interactions usually affect the system parameters, for which the thresholds are provided in BAN requirements. For example, the heat dissipation (un-intentional interaction) from the nodes affects the body temperature (system parameter). The modeling paradigm of BAND-AiDe hypothesizes that **any interaction of the computing unit with the physical world will take place within a bounded region**. Therefore, all interactions are limited within a region defined in the LCPS. To this effect, two types of regions for intentional and un-intentional interactions are specified in the physical unit. These regions are described below.

– The *region of interest (ROIn)*. This construct facilitates the modeling of the intentional interactions, e.g., the sensing and the wireless communication region. Each ROIn has two attributes.

  * A **monitored parameter**. This construct models the system parameters that are affected by the intentional interactions. For example, the physiological signal sensed by a worker node can be a monitored parameter, which is affected by the node's sensing capabilities (electromagnetic interaction, `http://www.quasarusa.com/`).

  * A **region boundary**. This attribute represents the limits of the bounded region, within which the intentional interactions are confined. The region boundary depends on the variation of the monitored parameters. For example, when the sensed signal is the monitored parameter, the sensing range of the worker node becomes the region boundary.

– The *region of impact (ROIm)*. This construct is used to model the un-intentional interactions. The ROIm consists of three attributes.

  * A **physical property**. This attribute characterizes the physiological parameters such as blood glucose level, blood pressure, and tissue temperature. These properties depend on the location of the node, physiological conditions, and environmental factors such as the temperature and pressure (`http://urwhatueat.org/carb5.html`).

  * The **physical dynamics**. This construct enables modeling of the physical processes. These processes are normally expressed in terms of complex equations. For example, the process of body-temperature variation is governed by a partial differential equation [59].

  * The **region boundary**. This is similar to the region boundary in the ROIn. However, the region boundary of the ROIm depends on the physical properties and dynamics. Since the physical dynamics is governed by differential equations,

the region boundary can be specified by boundary conditions on the equations. These conditions are generally limits on the physical properties outside the ROIm. For example, in the case of a temperature rise in the human body, it can be assumed that the body temperature is 37 °C outside the ROIm. These boundary conditions can then be employed with the associated differential equation [59] to obtain the region boundary.

- *Local interactions.* The local interactions are cyber-physical interactions between the computing unit and the physical unit within an LCPS (denoted by the dashed lines in Figure 4.6). The intentional and un-intentional interactions are modeled using the following constructs.
  - **Intended interactions.** These are modeled as transfer of information between the computing unit and the ROIn. For example, the sensing of physiological signals from the human body by a node can be modeled by this construct.
  - **Unintended interactions.** These interactions are modeled as transfer of energy between the computing units and the ROIm. For example, heat transfer from the computing unit to the corresponding ROIm can be modeled by this construct.

  Note that interactions between the ROIn and the ROIm of an LCPS are also defined. These are used for representing certain special cases, where there are inter-dependences between the ROIn and ROIm.

Interactions among the LCPSes. In the BAN-CPS model, interactions between different LCPSes can also take place. For example, the wireless communication between two sensor nodes in a BAN is a form of information transfer between two different LCPSes. This phenomenon can be modeled by introducing the concept of interconnections between the LCPSes. These interconnections are called *global interactions* (as depicted by the two-way dashed arrows in Figure 4.6). Global interactions between two LCPSes normally occur whenever there is an overlap in the ROIn or the ROIm of the two (as shown in Figure 4.7). This notion of global interaction facilitates the modeling of a network of nodes in a BAN (through overlapping of the ROIns) or of the cumulative thermal effect of the nodes on a particular area of the physical environment (overlapping of the ROIms). Global interactions can be intended or unintended due to the overlapping of the ROIns or ROIms of the interacting LCPSes, respectively.

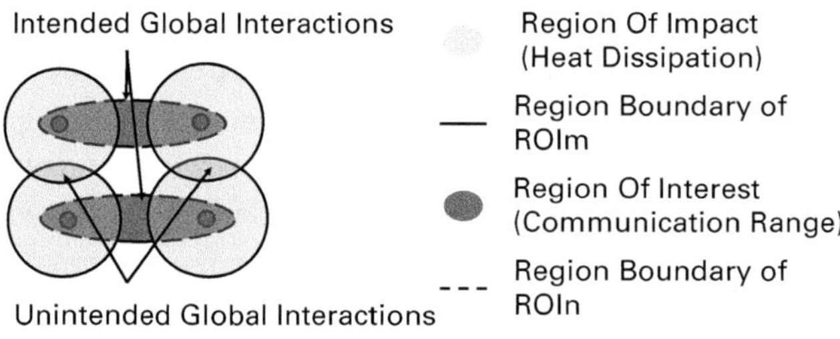

Figure 4.7   Global interactions.

Analysis-parameter modeling

Analysis of a model generally involves specific methodology to solve equations that govern the physical dynamics. The solution techniques often require a configuration, i.e., assigning values to certain specific parameters determining the quality of the solutions. For example, solving Pennes' equation will require the FDTD time-and-space-discretization approach. The granularity of such discretization can be specified in the model as sets of *constants*. Further, the aggregate functions can be specified as a set of equations combining the physical dynamics of different LCPSes.

4.4.2   The BAND-AiDe analyzer

The BAND-AiDe analyzer determines the BAN behavior from the BAN-CPS model. The behavior is then verified against the requirements given as input to the BAND-AiDe modeling framework. Figure 4.4 shows the work flow of the BAND-AiDe analyzer.

The models from the BAND-AiDe modeling framework are first parsed into a suitable format by a **model parser**. There are three different components of the parser: (1) the requirements parser, (2) the BAN-CPS parser, and (3) the analysis-parameter parser. These components correspond to the three modeling aspects of the modeling framework (Section 4.4.1). The output of the *requirements parser* is a set of constants indicating the thresholds on different system parameters. The *analysis parser* provides parameters (a set of constants) related to the analysis methodology (e.g., the configuration for equation solvers, the time step, and the spatial granularity). The *BAN-CPS parser* extracts the hierarchical organization of the BAN-CPS model in a structure using which interactions and aggregate effects can be computed. The outputs of the parsers are called the *model variants*.

The pseudocode of the analyzer is shown in Algorithm 4.1. The *EvaluatePhysicalProperty* and *EvaluateMonitoredParameter* routines evaluate the variations of the physical properties and monitored parameters within the region boundaries (denoted by RB) of the ROIm and ROIn of each LCPS, respectively. These evaluations essentially compute the local interactions within an LCPS. Note that the representation of the region boundary by the notation GCPS.LCPS(i).ROIm.RB reflects the hierarchical nature of the constructs (Figure 4.6). Similar notations are also used for the other constructs.

The next process is to identify and compute the interactions between different computing units. This process involves the computation of the global interactions. In the pseudocode, this is achieved by iterating through all n^2 possible pairs of LCPSes (where n is the number of nodes in the BAN) and checking whether the RBs of LCPS pairs overlap. These overlapping regions are tracked by the parameters IntFm and IntFn, for ROIm and ROIn, respectively. The aggregate variations of the physical properties and the monitored parameters are then evaluated for these regions of intersections. The aggregation functions provided in the analysis parameter model are used to this end.

After computing the interactions and aggregate effects, the analyzer checks the monitored parameters and the physical properties against the requirements. This process is called the requirements-verification process. The results of the verification process are compiled to generate an analysis report.

Process: **BAND-AiDe Analyzer (BAND-AiDeModel)**

Model Parser   /* Parse model and extract the Model Variants */
GCPS = Model Parser(BAND-AiDeModel.BAN-CPSModel);
[Performance Thresholds] = Requirements parser(BAND-AiDeModel.RequirementsModel);
[Analysis Parameters] = Analysis Parameter parser(BAND-AiDeModel.AnalysisParametersModel);

Interactions between computing unit and physical system
for each i from 1 ... n
    GCPS.LCPS(i).ROIm.Physical Property = EvaluatePhysicalProperty(GCPS.LCPS(i).ROIm, AnalysisParameters)
for each i from 1 ... n
    GCPS.LCPS(i).ROIn.Monitored Parameter = EvaluateMonitoredParameter(GCPS.LCPS(i).ROIn,
AnalysisParameters)

Interaction between different computing units
for each i from 1 ... n
    for each j from 1 ... n
        if GCPS.LCPS(i).ROIm.RB overlap with GCPS.LCPS(j).ROIm.RB
        IntFm(i,j) = 1;
        else
        IntFm(i,j) = 0;
        if GCPS.LCPS(i).ROIn.RB overlap with GCPS.LCPS(j).ROIn.RB
        IntFn(i,j) = 1
        else
        IntFn(i,j) = 0;
for each IntFm(i,j) == 1
    GCPS.LCPS(i).ROIm.Physical Property = Compute the aggregate effect in the intersecting region;
    GCPS.LCPS(j).ROIm.Physical Property = Compute the aggregate effect in the intersecting region;
for each IntFn(i,j) == 1
    GCPS.LCPS(i).ROIn.Monitored Parameter = Compute the aggregate effect in the intersecting region;
    GCPS.LCPS(j).ROIn.Monitored Parameter = Compute the aggregate effect in the intersecting region;

Requirements Verification
for each Param.time step
    for each Param.space step
        Compare Monitored Parameter with performance thresholds
Return Verification Results

Algorithm 4.1 Pseudocode for the BAND-AiDe analyzer. This encodes the processing
flow shown in Figure 4.4.

4.4.3   Implementation

Given the modeling framework and the analysis work-flow in the previous subsections,
this subsection presents the current implementation of BAND-AiDe. The modeling
framework of BAND-AiDe is developed using the Abstract Architecture Description
Language (AADL). AADL is an industry-standard language to model real-time embedded systems and is suitable for implementing BAND-AiDe for the following reasons.

- AADL specifications are hierarchical in nature, which helps in specifying the BAN-
  CPS model.
- AADL has dedicated constructs to model hardware and software of embedded computing devices. This will be helpful in modeling the behavior of the computing units
  in the BAN.
- AADL has been used to model wireless sensor networks [78]. This modeling is
  directly applicable for the BAN computing units.

```
system Component
  features
    INPUT: input type;
    OUTPUT: output type;
properties
    P1: property type;
end Component;

system implementation Component.imp
  subcomponents
    C1: component type;
    C2: component type;
properties
    P1: specific implementation;
annex
    A1: specific implementation;
connections
    connection between inputs and outputs of two subcomponents: connection type;
end Component.imp;
```

Algorithm 4.2 Component declaration and implementation.

- AADL provides facilities for language extension through development of annexes. These facilities can be used to incorporate the generic constructs of the BAN-CPS model in AADL.

AADL model specification is inherently hierarchical in nature in that the user develops a system as a congregation of components. Such a composite model is declared by the **system** keyword in AADL. Each system has two parts to its specification, as shown in Algorithm 4.2.

1. System declaration. This is the definition of the component that includes its inputs and outputs through which other components can communicate with it, denoted by the keyword **features**, salient properties of the component that characterize its behavior in the particular analysis, denoted by the keyword **properties**, and any functionality that the user wants to include which is not supported by AADL, denoted by the keyword **annex**. AADL has the provision for developing annexes where a user can implement customized specification rules and constructs to supplement the AADL specification language.

2. Component implementation, denoted by the keyword **implementation**. This is a specific instance of the declaration. In this part of the specification the subcomponents of the component are specified. The different subcomponents are interconnected through specific connection definitions, denoted by the keyword **connections**, in the desired manner to set up the model of the component. Specific values are assigned to the properties and annex variables of the component.

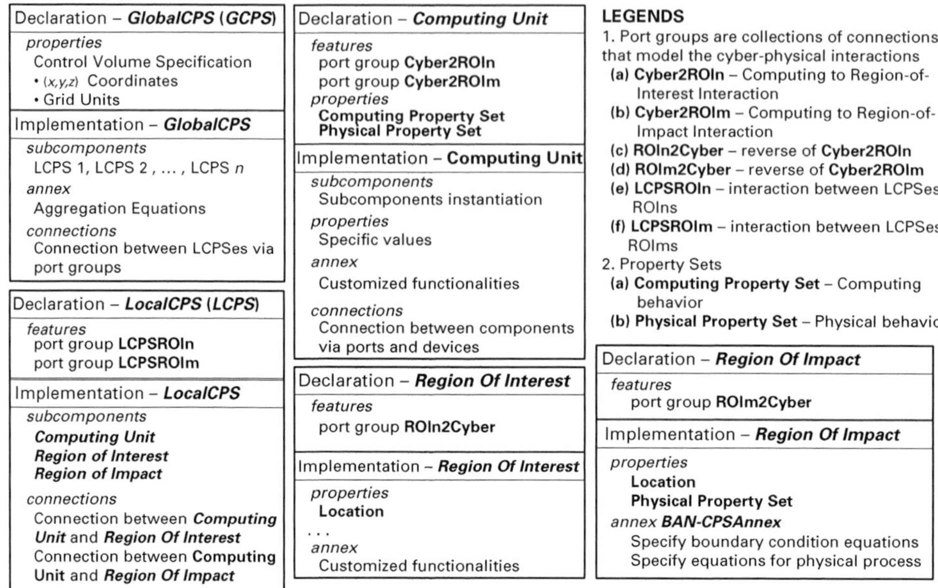

Figure 4.8   AADL specification of the BAN-CPS model.

Model specification

The GCPS in the BAN-CPS model (Figure 4.6) can be represented using the *system* construct in AADL (as shown in Figure 4.8) and is named **Global CPS (GCPS)**. In the GCPS, the monitored region of the human body is specified as a grid. The origin and the units of the grid are specified using the *properties* construct. The constants for the requirements specification and the analysis parameters can be provided in the GCPS specification using separate *property sets*, which are AADL constructs to specify system attributes. The **GCPS** consists of several *subcomponents* called **Local CPSes (LCPSes)**. These are also modeled using the *system* construct. Each **LCPS** consists of three *subcomponents*: (1) the **Computing Unit**, which models a single worker node, (2) the **Region of Interest**, which models the ROIn, and (3) the **Region of Impact**, which models the ROIm. The *system* construct is used to model these subcomponents. The **Computing Unit** has two *property sets*, the **Computing Property Set** and the **Physical Property Set**, to model its cyber and physical behavior, respectively. The **Computing Unit** can be modeled in a conventional way, containing *subcomponents* such as processor, memory, radio, and bus [78].

The location of the worker node is specified using the **Location** *property set*. This property set gives the coordinates of the worker node with respect to the origin and grid units defined in the GCPS. Within an ROIm, the worker node is considered to be the origin. The ROIm consists of properties from the **Physical Property Set**. The dynamics of the physical system which involves specification of complex analytic expressions is specified with the help of the **BAN-CPSAnnex**. This *annex* extends AADL with customized constructs for specification of partial differential equations. The **Region**

Boundary of the ROIm is represented by boundary conditions on the properties of the physical unit. A similar approach is taken to implement the ROIn of the LCPS.

The global and local interactions in the BAN-CPS model are specified with the help of the *port group* AADL construct. The port group construct is an assembly of different types of *port*s. These *port*s, together with their interconnection using the *connections* construct, model information transfer among the subcomponents. The **Computing Unit** has two *port groups*: (1) **Cyber2ROIn**, which specifies the *intended interaction* of the computing unit with the ROIn; and (2) **Cyber2ROIm**, which specifies the unintended interaction of the computing unit with the ROIm. The global interactions are modeled using two types of *port groups*, **LCPSROIn** and **LCPSROIm**, in each LCPS. These *port groups* signify interactions between a computing unit of an LCPS and the ROIn and ROIm of some other LCPS, respectively.

The analysis framework

The analysis of BAN models specified using BAND-AiDe is performed by a simulation framework developed in a high-level language such as JAVA. The analysis framework uses the parsers provided by the OSATE platform to parse the AADL constructs. Further, it uses the **BAN-CPSAnnex** parser for the customized differential-equation constructs. In the BAN-CPS Annex specific constructs can be declared for denoting differential equations. For example, the construct *DeltnXY* represents the mathematical operator $\delta^n X/\delta^n Y$. The differential equations are parsed using context-free grammars of the form

```
Operator = Variable * DeltnXY * Operator + Variable * Operator |
           Variable * DeltnXY * Operator - Variable * Operator | null
DeltnXY = Delt1XY | Delt2XY ................ Variable = any string
| null
```

The parsed differential equations are represented in the form of a parse tree. In the analysis plug-in, the parse-tree representation of the equations is converted into a mathematical form. At the time of writing, the BAN-CPS Annex converts the parsed equations into FDTD form, which can be solved using any FDTD solver. To this end, the analysis plug-in is integrated with domain specific tools such as MATLAB®. The analysis results are provided in a graphical format through MATLAB®.

4.5   Demonstrating design and analysis with BAND-AiDe

This section shows the usage of the BAND-AiDe tool to model and analyze BAN operations. For simplicity, thermal effects are considered for maximum node power consumption. Thermal-safety verification under this worst-case situation guarantees thermal safety in all other situations. To obtain the model parameters for BAND-AiDe through experimental evaluations, Ayushman was implemented in a BAN consisting of TelosB motes interfaced with temperature, humidity, and physiological sensors. The usage of the BAND-AiDe tool is demonstrated for (i) a *single medical device* and (ii) a *network of sensor nodes*, as summarized in Table 4.1 and described in the following subsections.

Table 4.1 BAND-AiDe usage for safety evaluations

Verification	Input	Model	Analysis

Safety and sustainability of a single wearable medical device (pulse oximeter)	**Requirements**
	Safety Threshold temperature T_{th} of the human body which should not be exceeded [83].
	Sustainability Device power consumption less than available power from scavenging sources.
	BAN system
	Single worker node consisting of a TelosB mote interfaced with the fingertip pulse-oximeter device deployed on the index finger. Scavenging sources are considered on the human body, which charge the nodes through inductive charge transfer.
	Analysis parameter
	Differential-equation-solver FDTD parameters (time step and space steps).
		Requirements model
		Requirement verification parameter T_{th}
		BAN model
		GCPS – 1 LCPS.
		LCPS – Computing Unit (CU) + ROIm + ROIn
		  CU – subcomponents + properties
		    subcomponents – LED, radio, processor, scavenging source
		    properties – power dissipation, temperature
		  ROIm – physical property + physical dynamics + region boundary
		    physical property – temperature
		    physical dynamics – Pennes' bioheat equation
		    region boundary – 30 mm by 30 mm square region
		  ROIn – charging range of the scavenging source
		Analysis parameter
		Time step and space granularity parameters of FDTD solver
			Safety
			Thermal map of the fingertip skin for continuous operation of the pulse oximeter is tested against safety threshold set by the requirements.
			Sustainability
			The power consumption of the device is compared against the available power from scavenging sources.

Safety evaluation of network of devices communicating securely	**Requirements** Safety Lower bound on the tissue temperature for the optimal cluster-head-selection sequence. Sustainability Budget on the available power from the energy-scavenging sources.	**Requirements model** Upper threshold T_{th} on the maximum temperature rise of the human tissue **BAN model** GCPS – n LCPSes LCPS – Computing Unit (CU) + ROIn + ROIm	**Safety** Each cluster-head-selection sequence is evaluated to compute the thermal map of the tissue.

BAN system

Network of worker nodes implanted within the human tissue. The worker nodes are interfaced with ECG sensors. Communication protocol is cluster-based [68], where several nodes form a cluster with a nominated cluster head. The cluster head collects data from all the cluster members and sends them to the wearable worker node. A cluster-head-selection sequence is specified, which denotes the order in which cluster heads are selected during the data-transfer process. The Ayushman health-monitoring application is executed on each node. The radio of each worker node can be turned off during different stages of their operation.

Scavenging sources charging the nodes via inductive charge transfer are assumed.

Analysis parameter

Cluster-head-selection sequence, differential-equation-solver FDTD parameters (time step and space steps).

Sensing rate, data-transmission rate, rate of PKA execution, time interval of observation.

CU – properties
  properties – power dissipation
ROIn – monitored property + region boundary
  monitored property – radio signal strength
  region boundary – communication range
  (intersection of ROIn indicates connectivity)
ROIm – physical property + physical dynamics + region boundary
  physical property – temperature
  physical dynamics – Pennes' equation
  region boundary – preset value
  (intersection of ROIm requires evaluation of cumulative effect)
LCPS – scavenging source + ROIn
  CU – properties
  properties – available power for scavenging source
ROIn – a worker node receives power from a scavenging source if it falls inside the ROIn

Analysis parameter

Cluster-head-selection sequence

Time step and space granularity parameters of FDTD solver

Data transmission time t_{TX}, Sensing time t_{S}, and PKA execution time t_{PKA}

Different cluster-head-selection sequences are compared based on the maximum temperature in the control volume.

Sustainability

24-h operation of the Ayushman application was considered, where sensing was performed at a rate of 60 samples per second, data communication every 5 seconds, and PKA operation once in 24 h.

4.5.1   Safety verification of a single wearable medical device

This section presents the safety verification for a single high-power wearable medical device. To this end, we assume the scenario in Example 4.4, where the medical device considered is a TelosB mote interfaced with a Smith fingertip pulse oximeter (PPG) device (http://www.smithsoem.com/) deployed on the index finger. The pulse-oximeter probe which is in direct contact with the human finger passes light at a particular intensity through the finger during its operation. The pulse rates are then derived from the modulations in the sensed light intensity. Power is consumed by the device to perform sensing, computation, and transmission.

BAND-AiDe inputs

The safety requirement input to BAND-AiDe is the upper threshold on the skin temperature, which is 39 °C as obtained from the Henriques–Moritz equation [83]. For sustainability, the requirement is to keep the power consumption of the device lower than the available power from the scavenging sources. Pennes' bioheat equation is used to characterize the thermodynamic processes. The thermodynamics of the finger involves heat-transfer mechanisms such as thermal conduction, convection, radiation, and electromagnetic absorption. The thermal-safety-analysis parameters include the time steps and space granularity (e.g., grid size, where a grid is the smallest volume of the human body within which the temperature is assumed to be constant) of the solvers for equations (in this case, Pennes' equation) describing the thermodynamic processes.

The BAND-AiDe model

The requirement and analysis parameter modeling involves representation of the skin temperature threshold, the available power from the scavenging sources, the scavenging duration, and the time steps and grid sizes (to solve Pennes' equation) as constants. For the BAN-CPS modeling, the GCPS is represented as a system with a single LCPS. The medical device is modeled as the computing unit, which has several subcomponents such as an LED array, a radio, and a processor. These subcomponents are the generic components of the pulse-oximeter device. Each subcomponent has a set of physical properties (such as power dissipation, operating temperature) that model its thermal characteristics. The ROIm models the thermodynamics of the human skin using Pennes' bioheat equation as follows:

$$\rho C_p \frac{dT}{dt} = K \, \nabla^2 T - b(T - T_b) + \rho \text{SAR} + P_c + A\sigma(T_r^4 - T^4), \tag{4.1}$$

where ρ is the mass density, C_p is the specific heat, K is the thermal conductance, T is the temperature of the skin, P_c is the power generated by any heat source (i.e., the device), A is the surface area of the radiating entity (i.e., the LED array in the case of the pulse oximeter), T_r is the surface temperature of the radiating entity, b is the blood perfusion constant, T_b is the blood temperature, and SAR is the specific absorption rate of the skin (i.e., the amount of electromagnetic radiation absorbed per unit volume of skin).

Table 4.2 Skin temperatures after eight hours of pulse-oximeter operation at different device temperatures (burn threshold 39 °C)

Device temperature (°C)	Maximum skin temperature (°C)
43.0	38.2
43.5	38.5
44.0	39.2
44.5	39.4
45.0	39.7

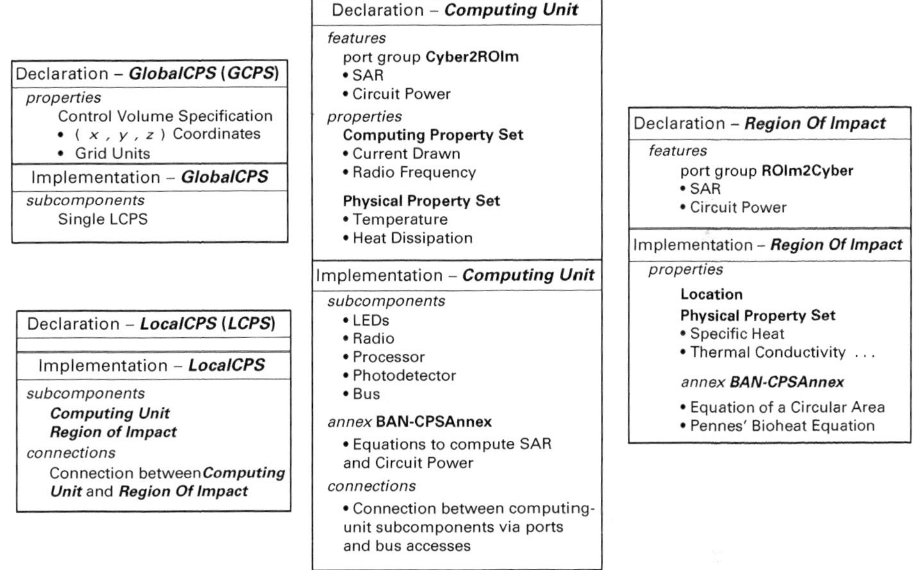

Figure 4.9   The AADL code structure for pulse-oximeter safety modeling.

The region boundary of the ROIn is preset to a 30 mm × 30 mm square region on the fingertip skin, which is the size of the pulse-oximeter probe (http://www.smithsoem.com/), which is in direct contact with the fingertip. The operating temperature of the pulse-oximeter probe is assumed to be constant [72]. This is because the typical BAN workload is highly repetitive (with a re-occurring cycle of sensing, computation, and transmission), which causes the probe temperature to reach a steady state quickly. Detailed BAND-AiDe implementation is shown in Figure 4.9. Given the inputs and the BAND-AiDe model, the BAND-AiDe analyzer performs the safety analysis employing the work-flow shown in Figure 4.4 and Algorithm 4.1.

Safety verification

The BAND-AiDe analyzer computes the temperature at different points on the skin by solving Pennes' equation using the FDTD approach. Table 4.2 shows the maximum skin temperature reached during the eight hours of operation of the pulse oximeter at different

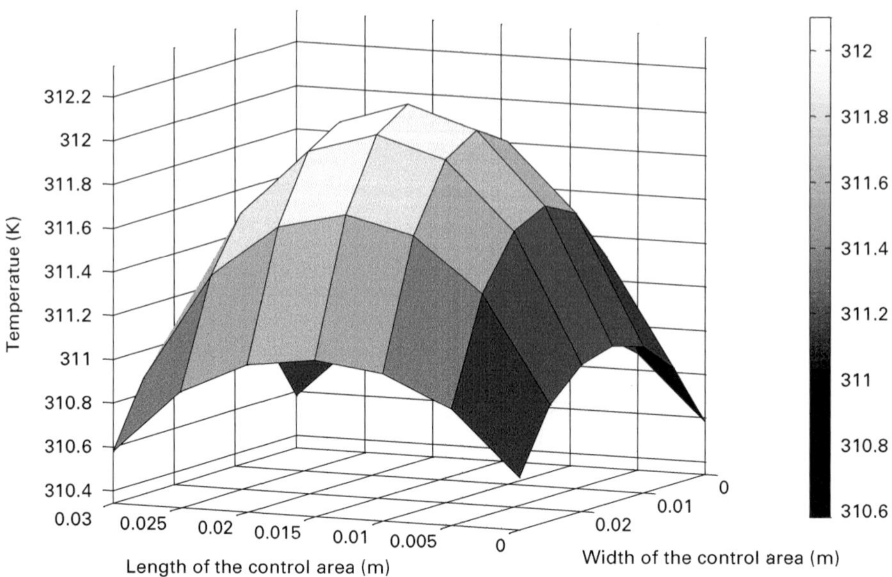

Figure 4.10 A thermal map of fingertip skin for 8 h of pulse-oximeter operation at 44 °C.

device temperatures. The AADL code structure is shown in Figure 4.9. A sample thermal map of the skin for a pulse-oximeter operating temperature of 44 °C is shown in Figure 4.10. It can be verified that the maximum temperature reached after eight hours of operation is 39.2 °C, which violates the thermal safety requirement. An experimental study performed on pulse-oximeter thermal safety [72] showed that blisters are observed in human skin when a pulse oximeter is operated continuously for eight hours at a device temperature of 44 °C. Our results concur with these experimental observations and are hence verified.

4.5.2 Safety verification of a network of devices

This section presents the safety verification for a network of sensor nodes. We consider the scenario in Example 4.3, where multiple sensors form a cluster-based network with the smart phone as the base station. Periodic changes in the cluster head are required in order to reduce the maximum tissue temperature during the communication operation.

BAND-AiDe inputs

As for the single-device verification in Section 4.5.1, the safety-requirement input for verifying the network of nodes is the upper threshold on the skin temperature, i.e., 39 °C. The analysis parameters corresponding to Pennes' equation are the same as in Section 4.5.1. The control volume was divided into 30 × 30 cells, where the cell size was set to 0.005 m. The aggregation function for the heat effect from multiple contributing nodes is provided as follows: (i) summation of the SAR values from the contributing nodes; (ii) summation of the power generated from the contributing nodes; and (iii)

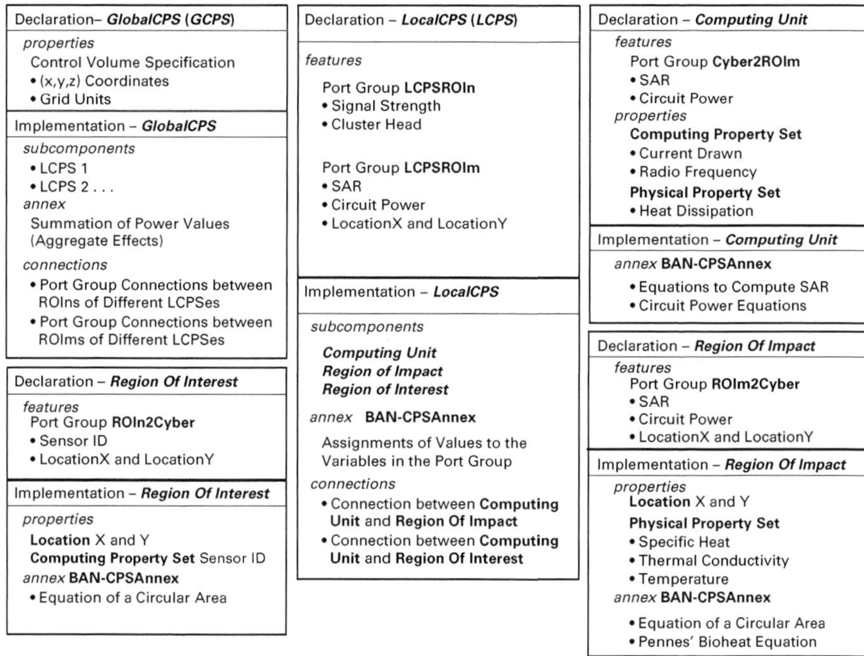

Figure 4.11 The AADL code structure for multi-hop-communication evaluation.

application of the summed SAR and generated power values in Pennes' equation (i.e., Equation (4.1)). In addition, the leadership sequence is input as an analysis parameter.

BAND-AiDe model

The GCPS consists of multiple LCPSes. The LCPS modeling for each worker node is the same as in Section 4.5.1. In addition, the ROIn of each LCPS models the communication range of the node. The intersections between the ROIns reflect the connectivity among the corresponding sensor nodes. The leadership sequence is represented as a string of constant integers. Details of the BAND-AiDe implementation are shown in Figure 4.11.

Safety verification

To evaluate the tissue temperature distribution, Pennes' bioheat equation is solved using the FDTD solvers (as in Section 4.5.1). This aggregate effect was calculated by summing up the heat contribution of each node to a particular grid, as described in Section 4.5.2. The power consumption of a leader worker node was 60 mW [84] while that of a non-leader worker node was 12 mW. This power consumption was experimentally measured for TelosB motes at 0 dB and −7 dB of radio attenuation, respectively. For a sample BAN cluster of 10 sensor nodes, the leaders were changed every second. Each leadership sequence was operated once for a short period of 1,000 s and then for a long duration of two days. Our results for 1,000 s of exposure match with the observations in [69]. Table 4.3 shows maximum tissue temperatures for different leadership sequences at different exposure times. The maximum temperature is below the safety threshold of 39 °C

Table 4.3 Tissue temperature rise for different leadership sequences (burn threshold 39 °C)

Leadership Sequence										Maximum tissue temperature (°C)	
										Exposure for 1,000 s	Exposure for 2 days
(5	2	8	6	1	7	3	4	10	9)	37.1145	37.1632
(5	7	4	1	6	10	8	2	9	3)	37.1130	37.1614
(1	6	9	10	2	7	5	4	3	8)	37.1124	37.1757
(5	7	1	9	10	8	4	2	6	3)	37.1130	37.1585

for all these cases. It can be seen from Table 4.3 that, for a short duration of exposure, a different leadership sequence does not have much effect on the tissue temperature rise. However, for longer durations, the temperature rise is significant (around 0.02 °C). This shows that for long-term operation of implanted networks of medical devices the leadership sequence plays an important role in thermal safety.

This section described a tool that uses architectural modeling of BAN and human physiology for safety verification. The following section will discuss how the safety can be verified using formal methods.

4.6   Formal models for BAN safety

As discussed in Section 4.3, any modeling techniques for BAN (including formal modeling) can characterize the spatio-temporal effects of cyber-physical interactions. The modeling framework in Figure 4.6, which was proposed in [85], is used for BANs to model them as cyber-physical systems. Interaction safety with respect to thermal effects of computation in the sensors is considered, and GCPS is used to model such scenarios. Given the GCPS models, two types of analysis are performed: (a) simulation on a given set of test cases and (b) formal model-checking analysis. For simulation purposes BAND-AiDe, as proposed in [85] can be used, employing GCPS as the modeling tool and a generic simulation analysis framework for the models.

For model-checking purposes, a novel formal model that captures the spatio-temporal cyber-physical interactions is necessary. Such formal models can be referred to as spatio-temporal hybrid automata (STHA). A formal model generally represents a system as a collection of states and a set of dynamic equations that define the evolution of the states. Traditionally a state is defined as a collection of variables (called state variables), which vary over time, and a set of ordinary differential equations, which govern this variation over time. However, in STHA, as shown in Figure 4.12, a state should represent the system properties and their variations at a particular time and space. The state variables in such a formal model should vary in a continuous domain in both time and space, and their variation should be governed by spatio-temporal partial differential equations. In a traditional formal model, the temporal variation of the variables results in events that cause transitions of the system from one state to another. However, in STHA, since the state variables vary over both space and time, the events causing state transitions can be spatio-temporal in nature.

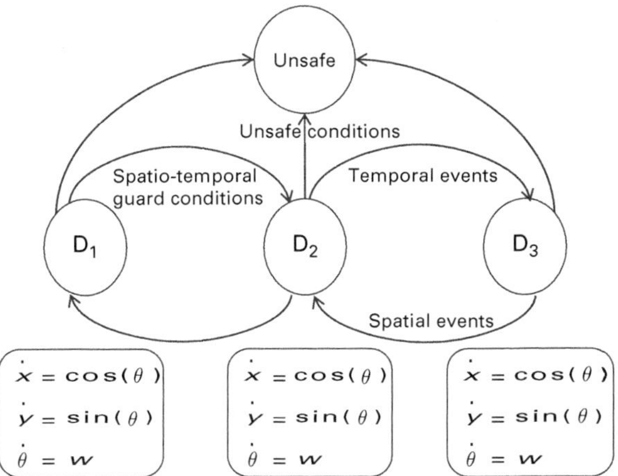

Figure 4.12   An abstract view of spatio-temporal hybrid automata.

An STHA model can be used for model-checking purposes for a CPS. One of the main analysis techniques for model checking is the reachability analysis. Reachability analysis can be used to perform safety analysis by marking a subset of states as *unsafe*. On performing reachability analysis, if those states are reached then the system operation can be concluded as *unsafe*. Current techniques to analyze hybrid automata [86] support system evolution in just one dimension (time). However, STHA require evolution in four dimensions. This not only renders the current available analysis tools inapplicable but also increases the complexity of the analysis. Reachability analysis for the STHA model can be performed by discretization of space and time dimensions. In this analysis, the continuous dynamics of the hybrid automata is evaluated by performing fixed-point computations of the specified equations. Then the discrete state transitions are simulated on the basis of the transition conditions to determine the states that can be reached from an initial state [86]. This can be done by setting an initial state and incrementing time, and then checking which states are reached as the continuous dynamics of the hybrid automata evolves.

4.7   Future research problems

Safety analysis for BANs is an important area that has been attracting increasing attention. The area of cyber-physical modeling of BANs requires more work. Physiological processes in the ROIm can affect the monitored parameters in the ROIn. Consider the example of an implanted sensor that measures physiological values from the human body and transfers them to a base station. Let the ROIn be defined as the communication range of the sensor, and let the ROIm be defined as the area of the surrounding tissue that receives thermal energy from the sensor due to its heat dissipation. Implantation often leads to growth of tissue around the computing unit, resulting in a change in the ROIm of the system [87]. However, this phenomenon leads to a change in the electromagnetic environment of the sensor, thus altering its communication capabilities or affecting the ROIn. Analysis of such scenarios is difficult due to the lack of models, and remains an open research problem.

The reachability analysis of STHA does not consider the time-varying dynamics and higher-order derivatives. For considering time-varying dynamics, Malisoff and Mazenc [88] suggested a novel reachability-analysis method using control-Lyapunov functions. The STHA analysis algorithm can be integrated with control-Lyapunov-function-based reachability analysis to achieve a comprehensive safety evaluation of the formal model.

Owing to discretization of the dimensions, errors will be introduced into the reachability analysis. In this regard, an important research objective is to ensure that *the approximation caused due to the discretization is an overestimation.* This discretization of the dimensions leads to approximations of the differential equations. Now in the analysis step there are two levels of approximations: (1) when three dimensions are discretized, whereupon the derivatives need to be approximated; and (2) when the differential equations are approximated during the reachability analysis in the remaining dimension. The characterization of the errors in the reachability analysis and proving the error bounds remains an open problem.

4.8　Questions

1. Why is safety important for BANs?
2. List the different safety categories for medical devices in BANs.
3. Create a taxonomy of different types of models for BAN safety analysis.
4. Why is model-based engineering preferred for safety analysis of BANs?
5. Model the thermal effects of a single-medical-device example using a finite-state machine (FSM). What are the difficulties in modeling with an FSM? Can you use hybrid automata to model the scenario? What are the difficulties?
6. Why do we need spatio-temporal modeling for BANs?
7. Provide your own examples (different from those mentioned in this chapter) to show spatio-temporal parameter variations in BANs.

5 Security

In this chapter, we focus on security for BANs. In particular, we present a new paradigm that uses environment coupling – a property inherent to BANs – for this purpose. However, before we delve into the details, we provide some general concepts and definitions pertaining to the notion of *security*, which we use throughout this chapter. Though the notion of security has many connotations, for the purposes of this book, we define it in the information-security context, as *preventing unauthorized entities from viewing, accessing, or modifying data generated within a system*. We use the term system in a generic sense to mean a computing system that takes an input, processes it, and provides an output.

In order to ensure information security within any system, five basic requirements need to be satisfied. (1) *Data integrity* ensures that all information generated and exchanged during the system's operation is accurate and complete without any alterations. (2) *Data confidentiality* ensures that all sensitive information generated within the system is disclosed only to those who are supposed to see it. (3) *Authentication* ensures that the system knows the identities of all the entities interacting with it, and vice versa. (4) *Authorization* ensures that any entity trying to access particular information from the system is able to access only that information to which it is entitled. (5) *Availability* ensures that any entity that uses the data and services and resources of the system is able to do so when required.

In order to secure a system, we need to have a clear understanding of the threats that affect it. A *threat* is a potential violation of security [89]. A system needs to be guarded against threats, in order to ensure its correct operation at all times. The execution of the threats is called an *attack*, while the entities which execute these threats are called *attackers* or *adversaries*. The common threats in the information-security context can be classified into three categories.

- *Eavesdropping*. Here, the attacker intercepts any information generated and communication within the system. It is a *passive attack*, i.e., the attacker does not interfere with the working of the system but simply observes its operation. Systems with communication capabilities are particularly susceptible to eavesdropping through traffic analysis. The confidentiality security property, which is usually enforced through some form of cryptographic encryption, ensures that such eavesdropping can be avoided.
- *Spoofing*. The attacker poses as a legitimate part of a system, and tries to take part in its operation. Once a spoofing attack has been mounted successfully, the attacker can

not only access information from the system, but also modify or delete it, in addition to introducing incorrect information. Spoofing can also result in incorrect execution of, and delay in provisioning of, specific services. At any point during the attack the system, being unaware of the deception, assumes all the data and services received from the attacker to be legitimate. Attack vectors such as man-in-the-middle are a variation of this class. Since the attacker interferes with the working of the system, it is an *active attack*. Authentication and authorization, together with confidentiality and integrity-protection properties, need to be enforced in order to avoid succumbing to this attack.

- *Denial of service.* The attacker inhibits the basic operation of the system. The attacks are active in nature and can be mounted, for example, by interfering with its functionality (e.g., jamming the communication channel), overwhelming it (e.g., by providing a bogus large input set to be processed, causing battery depletion or rejection of legitimate inputs), or through physical compromise (e.g., modifying the hardware/software of specific parts of a system, resulting in its inaccurate operation). The availability security property ensures that it can be avoided.

Given this high-level overview of the security requirements and threats to information security, in the rest of this chapter, information-security issues specific to the BAN context are discussed. Special focus is given to a novel environment-coupled security paradigm, and a detailed example is discussed, showcasing its capabilities.

5.1   The need for information security in BANs

One of the most important reasons to care about security in BANs is to prevent any form of unauthorized access and preserve *patient privacy*. The term *privacy* is defined as the ability to allow only the intended recipients to view a given item of information [90]. Privacy preservation is of particular importance in systems that collect health-related information. A person's health information is very sensitive in nature. Exposure of such information in an uncontrolled manner can lead to misuse, such as (1) deliberate alteration of health data of specific patients, leading to wrong diagnosis and treatment; (2) deliberate generation of false alarms or suppression of real alarms raised by the system in case of emergencies; and (3) economic and social discrimination against patients (e.g., insurance companies offering health insurance at high premiums to people who have certain chronic problems). With the electronic nature of data and wireless communication within BANs, the threats to patient privacy are much more severe than with the paper-based records of the past, which required manual access and were available at specific centralized physical locations only [11]. Therefore the ability of BANs to continuously collect, exchange, and store electronic medical data presents many avenues for abuses of privacy. Indeed, preserving patient privacy is also a legal requirement imposed by the *Health Insurance Portability and Accountability Act (HIPAA)* that mandates that all personally identifiable health information be protected [91]. Developing security solutions for privacy preservation in BANs is therefore of paramount importance.

Security in BANs is also important because of the potential to cause physical harm. BANs are often used in mission-critical applications such as health management. Often this requires actuation of some sort, usually in the form of drug delivery. This actuation capability makes them lucrative targets for hackers and tech-criminals. For example, there has been an attack on pacemakers that not only forced them to reveal a patient's electrocardiogram (ECG) data but also actuated untimely shocks [57]. Securing the actuation capabilities of BANs is therefore just as essential as privacy preservation. Additionally, the recent trend towards open design has led to the use of diverse completely off-the-shelf (COTS) components. Though this reduces the costs associated with building BANs, it also introduces complications for the system at large from a security standpoint. Different components of the system might be designed with different assumptions, and one needs to be very careful in integrating the components so as not to allow security vulnerabilities. Finally, there has been a growing trend towards integrating everyday items into the Internet, leading to the evolution of an "Internet of things." This will also extend to BANs. Indeed, the need to communicate the data to the back-end, usually a cloud, makes it inevitable. This is a considerable cause of concern insofar as it exposes the BAN to external influence.

The need for security solutions for BANs has been well documented [85, 91]. However, most BANs, considering their time-constrained *mission-critical* nature [92], are still designed solely to monitor health conditions with the goal of achieving data availability, efficiency, and self-configuration [85]. Any user (and the environment itself) is considered benign, and security is mostly dispensed with. Such an approach can have serious consequences, especially as the technology becomes more widespread. This peripheral treatment of security in BANs and other health-monitoring systems occurs because adding security tends to make the system (1) difficult to implement; (2) complex, which makes it difficult to manage and debug; (3) difficult to use for the patients and caregivers; and (4) expensive not only in terms of costs but also computationally and energy-wise [85]. However, considering security from the start of the system-design process and utilizing the inherent capabilities of the system can address many of these issues.

5.2   Securing a BAN as a cyber-physical system

This chapter focuses on enabling information security in BANs from a new perspective, that of cyber-physical systems (CPSes), which are environment-coupled in nature. This means that the cyber element takes many of its essential inputs from the physical environment in which it is placed. At the same time, it also controls the physical process through timely actuations. A BAN with its ability to monitor and act on the human body is a perfect example of such a system, which can be called a BAN-CPS. The involvement of the physical process introduces interesting possibilities and challenges in providing security for CPS. The principal focus of this chapter is the introduction and use of a new security approach for BAN-CPSes that is called *cyber-physical security* (CPS-Sec), which leverages the underlying physical process (i.e., the human body) to enable information security within the BAN. In the rest of the book we use the terms BAN and BAN-CPS interchangeably.

5.2.1   Securing BAN components

As discussed in Section 3.2, there are several modes of operation of a BAN as a CPS. However, most of the traditional security solutions have focused on the passive mode of operation of the BAN. Further, considering the current model of a BAN used for pervasive health monitoring (Figure 3.1), security is required at several levels as listed below.

- Communication between the sensors and the smart phone has to be secured since the data transmitted are sensitive physiological data.
- Communication between the smart phone and the cloud occurs through Wifi in a server–client manner, which needs to be secured.
- The physiological data are stored in several places, such as within the sensors, in the smart phone, and in the cloud. To ensure privacy, it is important to secure the storage.
- Access to sensitive data in the cloud has to be restricted to authorized personnel in order to maintain privacy.

Traditional security solutions are applied to all the above-mentioned privacy issues. For inter-sensor communication, cryptographic techniques such as probabilistic key-distribution schemes [93], master-key-based key-distribution schemes such as LEAP [94], and even asymmetric crypto-systems [95] have been proposed. Communication between the smart phone and the cloud is secured using Wifi Protected Access (WPA) or WPA2 encryption. Storage security using secret sharing and erasure coding has been proposed for sensors [96]. Moreover, for smart phones [97, 98] and clouds [99–101] storage security has been researched extensively. Access control of sensitive data has also been a strong focus of research among security engineers, and solutions that are based on access-control policies [102], role-based access control [103, 104], and criticality-aware access rules [105, 106] have been proposed.

Given the low computational capabilities of a sensor in the BAN, implementation of traditional security solutions is often infeasible and unusable. It often either requires storage and computation resources that are beyond the capacity of the sensors or blocks the execution of other applications in the sensor. In this chapter, we focus on how to leverage the cyber-physical interactions of the sensors with the human body to develop CPS-Sec solutions that are usable and feasible for implementation.

5.2.2   Challenges for CPS-Sec solutions

Applying CPS-Sec solutions is not straightforward. Some of the challenges in implementing them include the following.

- An *altered threat model*. The traditional threat model for computational systems has been focused solely on cyber threats. But the environment-coupled nature of CPS-Sec means that tampering with the physical environment around the CPS may result in its failure to function correctly. As an extension, attackers need not tamper with the environment itself, but can merely interfere with the sensing process, which might cause the CPS and its security apparatus to malfunction.
- *User-centric security*. The deployment of CPSes is not limited to specialized systems managed by tech-savvy people. Many of the applications of CPSes are systems in everyday use operated by non-technical people – medical monitoring systems, smart infrastructures, and so on. Therefore CPS-Sec solutions should have a high degree of usability, i.e., plug-and-play nature and security transparency – a characteristic that today's cyber-only security solutions largely lack.
- The *dynamism of the physical process*. One of the primary characteristics of CPS is that the behavior of the underlying physical process is not predictable. For example, in the case of the human body, a synchronously measured physiological signal produced at different locations on the human body will have significantly different correlation coefficients. CPS-Sec solutions with their dependence on physical processes have to compensate for this requirement.
- *Complexity*. CPS-Sec solutions may require the integration of primitives from multiple domains. This can potentially increase the complexity of the solution. The presence of bottleneck (low-capability) entities can exacerbate this problem and affect the timely execution of the security solution as well.

5.2.3　CPS-Sec solutions for BANs

In designing security solutions for BANs, one should consider not only the characteristics of the computational components involved (CPU, RAM, ROM, data rate), but also the interaction of the components with the physical process. More specifically, the idea is to use the monitoring capability of BANs to provide security. By utilizing this fundamental capability of BANs, security provision becomes intrinsically linked to the BAN operation and not something that is added later to a functioning system to protect it from threats. Another merit of CPS-Sec solutions is that they can now harness the complex and dynamic nature of the physical process provided by the human body for security purposes. Some of the principal characteristics of CPS-Sec solutions when used in BAN settings are as follows [11].

- *Usability*. Since BANs are closely linked to their environment, changes to the environment have a direct affect on the system, and this can be utilized in the security realm as well. Using environment characteristics as a basis for security primitives means that security overhead, deployment, and management abstractions need not be considered, freeing the designer to focus on functional aspects of the system.
- *Emergence*. CPS-Sec solutions are designed to provide the appropriate security functions such as confidentiality, integrity, and availability. However, they can also demonstrate additional "allied" properties, such as authentication of the BAN sensors.

As stated above, even though CPS-Sec solutions address many of the challenges of BAN security (especially the usability of security), their dependence upon the environment may make them susceptible to physical threats against BANs. However, this might not be a major point of concern for BAN-CPS, since the human body is one of the more secure environments in which sensors can be embedded. It is not easy to alter its functioning, at least in a surreptitious way. The same cannot be said about other domains where CPS-Sec solutions might be contemplated, for example power grids, where many substations are unmanned, and smart vehicles, which can be unmanned when parked. In this chapter, the use of CPS-Sec solutions for ensuring three of the fundamental security requirements/properties – confidentiality, integrity, and authentication – in BANs is discussed.

5.3   Traditional security solutions for BANs

Secure communication between any two entities is well understood and essentially has two phases: *trust establishment* and *data communication*. Trust establishment is a means of assuring each of the communicating entities that the other is legitimate. It is usually carried out through the establishment (and use) of cryptographic keys between the communicating entities [90]. Once the key has been established between two sensors, proving the presence of the key to the other entity establishes trust. For the purposes of this discussion we assume symmetric keys, without loss of generality. With trust established, data communication can now commence, which also utilizes the same key for maintaining the confidentiality and integrity of any data exchanged. Symmetric-key cryptography essentially involves the distribution of identical key strings at the entities that want to communicate with each other. That is, the same key is used both to encrypt and to decrypt a message, and all the entities that have access to the key can perform these operations. This is in contrast to asymmetric key cryptography, where each entity has a key pair. Data encrypted with one of the keys can only be decrypted by the other. The public-key infrastructure (PKI) is an example of asymmetric key cryptosystems, and it is usually much more expensive than the symmetric case.

5.3.1   Application of traditional approaches to key distribution

Key establishment (also referred to in the literature as key distribution or agreement) between sensors is therefore one of the most important aspects of secure communication between sensors. Traditional (environment-coupled) symmetric key-distribution schemes (e.g., sensor networks) can be classified into three generic categories.

- *Solely pre-deployment-based.* These techniques require the storage of a large set of keys in each sensor before deployment. Pre-deployment can be accomplished in a deterministic manner if the physical deployment details are known. For example, each node shares a pair-wise key with all its neighbors, a group key for multicasting to its neighborhood, and a network-wide key, to meet its communication requirements. Prominent examples include [93, 107–110].

- *Communication-based.* These techniques require some form of communication between entities in the network for key distribution. Such schemes either obtain keys from a central entity like the base station or require the exchange of information, such as random numbers or node IDs, which, together with a pre-deployed *master key*, is used for generating the shared key. Examples include [94, 111, 112].
- *Asymmetric cryptography-based.* These techniques use a pair of related keys (public and private) together with mathematically complex and computationally intensive algorithms to distribute symmetric keys between sensors. Prominent examples include [95, 113].

It can be seen that each of these protocol classes assumes some form of *pre-deployment*, which itself requires an underlying assumption of trust. This pre-deployment acts as an initial source of trust and forms the basis for distributing the actual key to be used in secure communication between sensors. However, this assumption makes them unsuitable for BANs. The main reasons for this stem from the following insecurities and hindrances to usability which are associated with pre-deployment.

- If the pre-deployment takes place at the factory where the sensors are manufactured, then hosts cannot trust the keys unless the entire key-distribution chain from the factory to the host is secured [114].
- If the pre-deployment is to be executed by the host, it would require them to make important decisions about the keys to be used. This might result in poor-quality keys, adversely affecting the security of the system.
- With pre-deployment, adding or moving nodes within the network would require additional host involvement. For example, if a node were added to the network, all the nodes in the neighborhood would have to have their keys updated.
- With pre-deployment, it is very difficult to change the keys in the network which have been compromised.

Over the years some solutions for secure pre-deployment have been proposed, such as Message in a Bottle [114] and Resurrecting Duckling [115]. These techniques require the presence of additional equipment (a Faraday cage) or extra communication interfaces on the sensors for a side-channel key deployment (e.g., infra-red, ultra-sound), and, more importantly, these techniques rely on considerable user involvement – making them unsuitable for BANs. Public-key cryptography, on the other hand, works slightly differently. It does not require any key pre-deployment, which is ideal for BANs; however, the principal problem comes in trust establishment itself, since there are no secrets between entities. Additional authentication mechanisms are needed in order for this to work, which may require host involvement, making the behavior akin to that of the pre-deployment-based scenarios discussed above.

Biometrics-based authentication schemes [116] have also been proposed for access control and ensuring privacy in BANs used for pervasive health care. In biometrics a template of some physiological characteristic of a person is maintained as a signature.

In subsequent authentication executions the same physiological characteristic is sampled and matched with the signature. A perfect match authenticates the user to the systems and grants him access. However, given the low computational capabilities of a sensor in a BAN, the implementation of traditional security solutions such as biometrics is often infeasible.

Further, as BANs become more commonly accepted and come to be worn by people with no chronic ailments, for preventive or non-medical applications, the overhead imposed by pre-deployment – in terms of security, user involvement, and general network management – will adversely affect the **usability** of the system. We therefore need a forward-looking security solution that follows the "plug-and-play" paradigm, is transparent and easy to use, and not only meets today's needs but is also flexible enough to be used in the future.

5.4   Physiological-signal-based key agreement (PSKA)

In order to make security protocols more usable, a CPS-Sec solution known as *physiological-signal-based key agreement* (PSKA) has been developed. It takes a fundamentally different view of security by *combining signal processing with cryptographic primitives*. It enables automated key agreement between sensors in the BAN without any form of user involvement by utilizing specific physiological stimuli from the human body.

The PSKA scheme is designed to establish a secure unicast channel between sensors in a BAN, and essentially works in five phases. (1) The two communicating sensors measure a pre-agreed physiological signal. (2) The sampled signal is processed and features are extracted from it, which are then quantized into a binary string. (3) One of the two nodes (designated the sender) then uses an arbitrary key to secure (encrypt/integrity-protect) any data it wants to communicate. (4) It then hides the key using this binary representation of the physiological signal feature, and transmits both the hidden key and secured data as a single message. (5) The receiving node retrieves the arbitrary key using the local version of the physiological signal, and checks it by verifying (decrypting/checking integrity) the data received. Once these steps have been executed, any subsequent secure communication between the sensors can take place without explicit physiological signal measurement using the key that they have just exchanged (except in special cases, for example if the network is being re-configured).

The scheme derives its security from the observation that the physiological-signal features generated from a subject are unique at any particular time. An adversary who is not in contact with the host's body will not be able to accurately measure the physiological signal and therefore cannot influence the secure communication taking place between the sensors. PSKA's *environment-coupled* key agreement means that nodes do not require any additional keying material in order to secure inter-sensor communication. Sensors can now be strapped on by a patient to ensure secure communication, in a *plug-and-play* manner. By extension, PSKA also allows one to add, move, or remove nodes without having to re-key large sections of the network.

5.4.1   Physiological signals: issues and properties

In order to understand the implementation of the PSKA protocol, we need to first understand in some detail the principal issues involved in utilizing physiological signals for enabling secure communication in BANs. A comprehensive discussion on some of the common physiological signals monitored and processed by BANs is given in Chapter 7. The first question is, of course, which physiological signal to use. The list of physiological signals generated by the human body is enormous; defining the criteria for choosing a physiological signal is therefore very important. Once the signal has been chosen, it has to be measured – sampled – at both of the sensors. Many issues exist in this regard, including synchronization of measurements, processing of the data collected, and reconciling the inherent difference in signals measured at different parts of the body. Once the measurement has been completed, the signals are processed to generate features that are then used for the key-agreement process. We describe each of these issues in detail below.

> *Choice and measurement.* The human body produces many physiological signals as a result of its "operation." Physiological signals, if they are to be useful for secure key agreement, need to have the following properties. (1) *Length and randomness*: the keys agreed upon are long and random to prevent brute-forcing. (2) *Low latency*: the duration of physiological signal capture required is minimal. (3) *Distinctiveness*: knowing the feature derived from the current value of the physiological signal of one subject will not provide significant advantage in guessing the keys being agreed by sensors on another host. An important characteristic of distinctiveness is that it authenticates the communicating sensors by ensuring that only sensors on the same BAN can agree on a shared key. (4) *Temporal variance*: knowing the physiological signals at any time will not provide significant advantage in determining the keys agreed upon in future executions of the scheme. Identifying physiological signals that possess the properties specified above is an important step in implementing PSKA. Table 5.1 shows some of the common physiological signals and their value range.
>
> *PSKA and biometrics.* Note that PSKA is fundamentally different from traditional biometric systems because the physiological-signal-based features used by it

Table 5.1 Ranges of common physiological signals, albeit unusable for PSKA

Physiological parameter	Range
Blood glucose level	64–140 mg/dl (varies with activity)
Blood pressure	120–160 mmHg (systolic) (range is from hypotension to hypertension)
Temperature	97.0–105.0 °F (range across ages and normal and abnormal conditions
Hemoglobin count	12.1–17.2 g/dl (varies between male and female, and depends on age and altitude)
Blood flow	>0.9 ABI (normal), <0.5 ABI (abnormal)

exhibit both distinctiveness and temporal variation. Biometric systems possess only the former, and actually depend on not possessing the latter. A biometric template created using a person's fingerprint, for example, is used for all subsequent authentication attempts made by the subject. The success of the authentication is based on the closeness of the match between a fingerprint sample, presented by the subject, and the original template. This model of operation allows an arbitrary amount of time to pass between two biometric measurements, since the biometric template itself is invariant. However, in the case of PSKA, physiological-signal features are time-variant. In order to be successful, the key-un-hiding process at the receiver requires synchronized measurements of physiological-signals with the sender. An attacker knowing the physiological-signal-based features at any given time has no advantage in compromising any past or future key agreements between sensors, a property that biometric templates do not possess.

Topographic specificity. Another important issue to be considered with physiological signals is the topographic specificity of the human body. That is, a given physiological signal appears to have similar trends but not exactly the same values when measured at different parts of the body [117]. As a result, the information symbols in the keys get re-ordered, leading to translational and rotational errors [118], which produce drastically different values. To overcome this problem of differences in the value of physiological signals, Cherukuri *et al.* [119] proposed treatment of the differences as analogous to the introduction of error while transmitting data between communicating sensors. The choice of error-correction mechanism is an important issue that needs to be considered carefully.

Physiological signal processing. One of the important properties of physiological signals is that they are time-variant and vary unpredictably. This prevents malicious entities from guessing the current value of the physiological signals or knowing future values if the current value is known. But this temporal variation also poses problems for the sensors trying to use the physiological signal to communicate securely. It is therefore necessary to ensure that the communicating sensors see identical (barring the topographic specificity) copies of physiological signals. A very important question in this regard is what kind of synchronization is required for PSKA? This will, of course, depend upon how the physiological signals are processed.

Signal processing of physiological signals can be done in two ways: through a *time-domain* or *frequency-domain* analysis. Time-domain-analysis signal values are directly quantized into binary streams and concatenated. However, due to the variation of physiological signals with time, the time-domain analysis tends to generate different features if the communicating sensors are not synchronized. To estimate the synchronization required for time-domain analysis, ECG and PPG data from the MIT PhysioBank MIMIC database (http://www.physionet.org/physiobank/database/mimicdb/) were used. For the 11 patients considered (those for whom the ECG and PPG data were available and complete), the average time difference between an ECG peak and the corresponding PPG peak was found to be $\mu = 250$ ms, with a standard deviation of $\sigma = \pm 6$ ms. Given the capability of sensor-synchronization protocols [36] to attain synchronization to within a few microseconds, for measuring the inter-peak interval only a relatively loose synchronization between the communicating sensors is needed. Note that different physiological signals will have different synchronization requirements. If the ECG were to be directly used, the level of synchronization would be limited by the sampling rate (f).

A frequency-domain analysis, on the other hand, tends to produce similar values even if the synchronization between the sensors is very loose. The experiments (see Section 5.4.4) show that even a difference of 1 s in measurement start times does not have any adverse effects on PSKA for PPG and ECG signals. However, converting the time-domain signal into a frequency-domain signal requires mathematical transforms that can be expensive.

5.4.2 PSKA protocol execution

The purpose of *physiological-signal-based key agreement (PSKA)* is to *facilitate secure inter-sensor communication* between two sensors by enabling them to agree upon a pair-wise symmetric key, using physiological-signal-based features. Figure 5.1 shows the complete process. A major challenge in implementing the error-correction approach

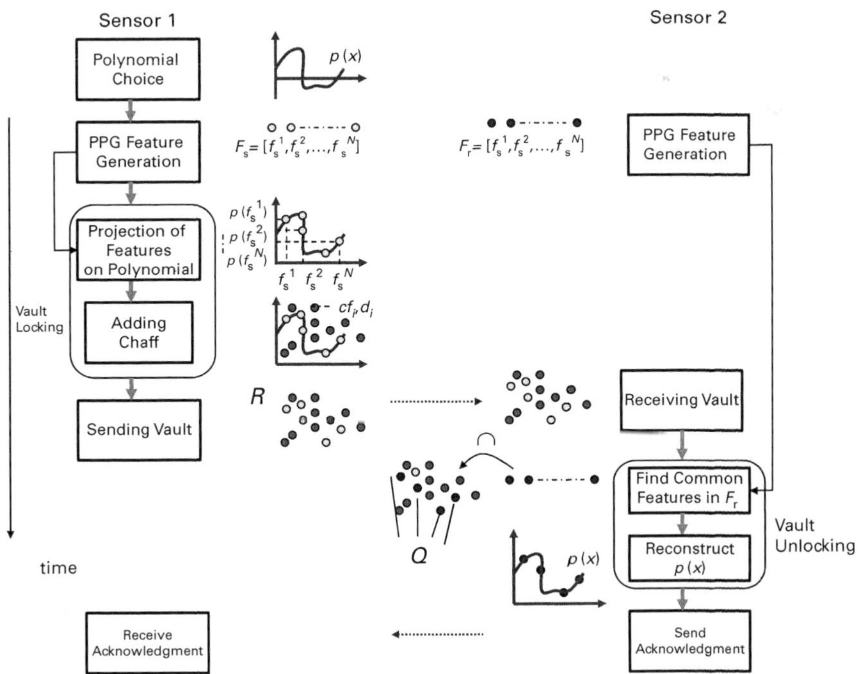

Figure 5.1 Key agreement in a BAN using PSKA.

described above is identifying the error-correction technique which can be used to correct the difference in physiological signals. The error-correction functions should be able not only to correct for the presence of a few differences in feature vectors, but also to handle re-ordering of, or the presence of, additional features (in one of the sensors) in the feature vector [118]. One of the ways of addressing this problem is by using a cryptographic construct called a *fuzzy vault* [118].

The fuzzy-vault scheme first proposed in [118] is designed to lock (hide) a secret (S) in a construct called a *vault* using a set of values A. Once the vault has been locked, it can be unlocked only with another set of values B that has a *significant* number of values in common with set A. The construction and locking of the vault is done by (1) generating a vth-order polynomial p over the variable x that encodes the secret S; (2) computing the value of the polynomial at different values of x from set A and creating a set $R = \{a_i, p(a_i)\}$, where $1 \leq i \leq |A|$; and (3) adding to R a randomly generated set of points called *chaff* that do not lie on the polynomial. Once the vault has been constructed, unlocking it using the set B is done by constructing a set $Q = \{(u, v)|(u, v) \in R, u \in B\}$. The unlocking process is possible only if Q has a significant number of legitimate (non-chaff) points that are on the polynomial [118].

Example 5.1. Let the polynomial be $p(x) = x + 1$, set $A = \{1, 2, 3\}$, and set $B = \{1, 3, 4\}$, then the vault R created by computing the polynomial's value at each point in A is $R = \{(1, 2)(2, 3)(3, 4)(4, 7)(6, 9)(7, 12)(8, 5)\}$. The last four points are the chaff points which do not fall on the polynomial. To unlock the vault the set Q is constructed, where $Q = \{(1, 2)(3, 4)(4, 7)\}$. Since the set Q has two points on the polynomial, it can be used to easily reconstruct the first-order polynomial and thus unlock the secret.

The use of polynomials ensures that the sets A and B need not have any order to them as long as they have a significant number of common values. The presence of the chaff points adds security to the vault, by hiding legitimate points and the actual polynomial. Unless the adversary knows a large number of points on the polynomial, it cannot reconstruct the polynomial.

We now discuss the fuzzy-vault scheme for key agreement in PSKA. This scheme can be mapped onto PSKA by setting the physiological-signal features obtained at one of the sensors to set A and those obtained at the other to set B, and generating a polynomial whose coefficients form the secret key that needs to be agreed upon. We use the terms *sender* for the sensor which creates the vault and locks it and *receiver* for the sensor that unlocks the vault to access the secret key. The key agreement occurs in seven steps.

Feature generation. First, both the sender and the receiver obtain physiological-signal-based features. This is a four-step process. (1) Both of the sensors sample the physiological signal in a loosely synchronized manner, at a specific sampling rate for a fixed duration. (2) The samples are divided into windows, and a fast fourier transform (FFT) is then performed on each of these parts. (3) The FFT coefficients of each of the overlapping windows (a pre-defined number of contiguous-signal time-series points) are then passed through a peak-detection function (a simple local-maxima detector) that returns a tuple of the form $\langle k_x^i, k_y^i \rangle$, where k_x^i is the FFT point at which a peak is observed (the peak location on the x-axis, also called the *peak index*), k_y^i is the corresponding FFT coefficient value (the magnitude of the peak, or *peak value*), and i is the index of the peak. The number of peaks observed by a sensor varies depending upon the situation. (4) These peak-index (k_x) and peak-value (k_y) pairs are quantized, converted into a binary string, and concatenated ($[k_x|k_y]$) to form a *feature*. Individual features obtained from a single measurement are grouped together to form a feature vector $F_D = \{f_D^1, f_D^2, ..., f_D^N\}$, where $f_D^l = [k_x^l|k_y^l]$, D is either the sender (s) or receiver (r) node, and N is the size of the feature vector, i.e., the number of indexes for which peaks were observed. The values of the different parameters used for feature generation are dependent upon the physiological signal used, and they need to be tuned during deployment. FFT peaks are chosen as features for two reasons: (1) they are simple to detect and (2) they allow us to overcome the topographic specificity since the frequency components of physiological signals measured at the same time on the same person are highly correlated. This enables us to use the FFT-based features to distinguish between sensors that are in the same BAN and those which are in different BANs, thus providing an efficient authentication mechanism and a basis for key agreement (see Section 5.4.4 for more details). At the end of the feature-generation process, the sender and receiver possess feature vectors of the form $F_s = f_s^1, f_s^2, ..., f_s^N$ and $F_r = f_r^1, f_r^2, ..., f_r^N$, respectively.

Polynomial choice. Once the features have been generated, the sender generates a vth-order polynomial of the form $p(x) = c_v x^v + c_{v-1} x^{v-1} + \cdots + c_0$, where the values of the coefficients (c_i) are selected randomly (using a pseudo-random-number generator, for example). The order of the polynomial (v) used within the BAN is not a secret; it is known to all sensors in the network. The coefficients, concatenated together, form the secret key that the sender wants to communicate to the receiver ($Key = c_v|c_{v-1}|...|c_0$). The length of this *Key* can be set to 128 bits (longer keys can easily be used), and, depending upon the order of the polynomial used, the coefficients can be obtained by dividing the *Key* accordingly.

Vault creation. With the polynomial and feature vector available, the sender now creates the fuzzy vault, by computing the set $P = \{f_s^i, p(f_s^i)\}$, where $f_s^i \in F_s$, and $1 \leq i \leq N$. It also computes a much larger set of M random chaff points of the form $C = \{cf_j, d_j\}$, where $cf_j \notin F_s$, $d_j \neq p(cf_j)$ and $1 \leq j \leq M$. Each chaff point, cf_i, is within the same range (0–2^{13}) as that of the features. Therefore, 2^{13} is the bound for the total number of points in the vault ($|R|$), which is equal to $|M| + |N|$. Let the cardinality of the set R denote the *vault size*.

Vault locking. The sender then randomly permutes the values in the vault $R = RandPermute(P \cup C)$, to ensure that the chaff points and the legitimate points are indistinguishable. The cardinality of the set C can vary with respect to the level of security needed. The larger the set C, the more difficult it is to break the vault. Section 5.4.4 discusses the relationship between the vault's size and its security in more detail. This set R is essentially γ from the conceptual overview.

Vault exchange. The sender communicates the vault R to the receiver using the following message: *Sender $\rightarrow$ Receiver : IDs, IDr, R, No, MAC(Key, R|No|IDs)*. Here, *IDs* and *IDr* are the IDs of the sender and receiver, respectively, *No* is a nonce (unique random number) for transaction freshness; *MAC* is a message authentication code (e.g., HMAC-SHA1); and the key (*Key*) used is the one that is being locked in the vault.

Vault unlocking. The receiver upon receiving the vault R first computes the set Q, where $Q = \{(b, c)|(b, c) \in R, b \in F_r\}$. It then tries to reconstruct the polynomial p from the points in Q using the Lagrangian interpolation (as suggested in [120]), according to which knowledge of $v + 1$ points $\{(x_0, y_0), (x_1, y_1), ..., (x_v, y_v)\}$ on a polynomial allows the reconstruction of a vth-order polynomial by performing the following linear combination: $p'(x) = \sum_{j=0}^{v} y_j d_j(x)$, where $d_j(x) = \prod_{i \neq j, i=0}^{i=v} (x - x_i)/(x_j - x_i)$. For the receiver to be successfully able to unlock the vault, the condition $|Q| > v$ should hold. It then takes $v + 1$ points (from Q) at a time and tries to unlock the vault. The coefficients of the resulting polynomial are then used to verify the MAC. This not only confirms the correctness of the unlocking process, but also authenticates the sender to the receiver (i.e., confirms that the sender is on the same BAN as the receiver). This works because of the distinctiveness and temporal variation of the physiological-signal features, which ensure that (1) the features generated from physiological signals for PSKA are drastically different for two different people and (2) the old vaults cannot be replayed since the features would have changed by that time, and cannot be unlocked (see Section 5.4.4 for more details).

Vault acknowledgment. If the unlocking was successful, the receiver then sends a reply back to the sender to inform it of its correct unlocking of the vault using the following message: *Receiver* $\rightarrow$ *Sender* : *MAC(Key, No|IDs|IDr)*. The symbols have the same meaning as above. The successful verification of the acknowledgment authenticates the receiver to the sender. This is because only a node on the BAN (receiver) which measured the same physiological signal at the same time as itself could have unlocked the vault, given the distinctiveness and temporal variation of the physiological-signal-based features. Section 5.4.4 provides more details on how these two properties are met.

We refer to the execution of these seven steps as an *iteration* of PSKA. The random key (*Key*) generated in the first step can be used to enable confidential, authenticated, and integrity-protected communication between sensors in a *plug-and-play manner, making BANs more usable*. Further, with PSKA, no random key or physiological features are ever reused. This ensures that knowledge of past keys or physiological features of a host cannot be used for subverting the vault (due to their temporal variation). Once the PSKA has successfully been executed, both the sender and the receiver have the common random *Key*. In order to use this key for future data communication, new data communication keys are derived, as suggested in [112], one at the sender $K's = f(Key, 1)$ and another at the receiver $K'r = f(Key, 2)$ to minimize the effects of cryptographic attacks on secured data communication; here f is a pseudo-random function.

5.4.3   Security of PSKA

Security issues in PSKA arise primarily due to its vault-exchange requirement. An eavesdropper can record the vault and try to construct the hidden polynomial (key) from it. In this section, we discuss the security implications of the two principal aspects of PSKA: the vault and its exchange.

Vault security. The use of the fuzzy-vault construct in PSKA ensures that, even though the two sensors might not have all features in common, they can still agree upon a common key in a secure manner. The security of the PSKA scheme is based on the difficulty of polynomial reconstruction. The hiding of the legitimate feature points among a much larger number of bogus chaff points, whose values are in the same range, makes the job of identifying the legitimate points very difficult. An adversary who does not know any legitimate points (since he or she cannot measure the relevant physiological signals from the host's body) has to try out each of the $v+1$ points in set R in order to be able to arrive at the correct polynomial. By the same reasoning, the greater the number of features an entity is aware of, the easier it is to reconstruct the hidden polynomial. An example is the receiver who has to try out $v+1$ points from the set Q in order to arrive at the correct polynomial. It needs to be pointed out that recent years have seen the development of remote-physiological-monitoring technologies [121, 122]. Such technologies in their current state are designed to work in a controlled environment and are susceptible to interference by objects in the environment, directionality, and motion artifacts. The use of such a technology to measure physiological signals in open environments and thereby compromise PSKA is an open issue that merits further investigation.

The strength of the vault is determined by the number of combinations an adversary has to try in order to find $v + 1$ legitimate points in the vault. For ease of understanding, this computation requirement is represented in terms of its equivalence to brute-forcing a key of a particular length (in bits). As expected, increasing the number of chaff points increases the security provided by the vault. The higher the order of the polynomial, the more common features are required for brute-force key determination and therefore the higher the security. Note that PSKA guarantees successful unlocking of the vault as long as the number of common features in Q is greater than v. By choosing the order of the polynomial to be a value $|F_s \cap F'_r| < v < |F_s \cap F_r|$, where $|F_s \cap F'_r|$ is the number of common features between feature vectors of two different individuals and $|F_s \cap F_r|$ is the number of common features between feature vectors for the same individual, successful vault unlocking can be ensured for the receiver but not for the adversary. Of course, this will work only if there is a discernible difference in the number of features between physiological signals collected from the same individual and those collected from different individuals. More on this in Section 5.4.4.

Choosing vault parameters is a balancing act between multiple criteria: the number of chaff points, feature length, and number of common features. The number of chaff points should be as large as possible relative to the total feature length within what can be tolerated by the system. A vault with an overwhelming number of chaff points is difficult to compromise by a pure brute-force attack. This, together with an appropriate polynomial order depending upon the common feature statistics, will ensure that the vault is secure.

Exchange security. The vault-exchange and acknowledgment phases make it very difficult for adversaries to know the key being agreed upon, for the following reasons.

- The presence of *IDr* in the vault-exchange message tells the sensors in the vicinity of the sender who the intended receiver is. The nonce *No* is used to maintain the freshness of the protocol, i.e., to ensure that the acknowledgment received is in response to the latest transmission.

- If a malicious entity sends a vault-exchange message (by replaying previous exchanges or creating its own vault using old physiological features), it will be discarded by any receiver because the MAC would not match due to a difference in the *Key* used, given the temporal variation of the physiological features.

- The vault has a number of chaff points many orders of magnitude greater than the number of legitimate points (for example, 1,000 chaff points to 30 legitimate feature points), which makes it difficult for adversaries to know which points are legitimate and which are not (as discussed above). A malicious entity that cannot unlock the vault cannot send a valid acknowledgement, since it would have to generate a valid MAC without the *Key*.

- A malicious entity trying to mount a man-in-the-middle attack has to be aware of the physiological-signal features being used. Without them, any modification of the vault during exchange would be caught because none of the $\binom{|Q|}{v+1}$ keys unlocked by the receiver will verify the MAC.

Thus we can see that PSKA meets all the security requirements enumerated earlier: it keeps the key agreement confidential (using the vault), integrity-protected (with the MAC), and authenticated (successful unlocking of the vault shows that the receiver is on the same BAN; more details will be given in the next section).

5.4.4   PSKA prototype implementation

In this section, we discuss how PSKA meets the required properties for key-agreement protocols in BANs. A proof-of-concept benchmark implementation of PSKA using MATLAB was reported in this regard.

Measuring physiological signals. The PSKA approach was validated using two of the most common physiological signals which can be collected from a person, namely the photoplethysmogram (PPG) and electrocardiogram (ECG). The former is a measure of the volumetric change in the distension of arteries due to the perfusion of blood through them during a cardiac cycle, while the latter is the representation of a host's cardiac cycle generated by the electrical activity of the heart. The PPG data utilized for analysis were collected from 10 volunteer subjects. Each volunteer was asked to sit upright with their hand firmly placed on a desk; an oximeter sensor was placed on the index finger of each hand. In the experiments it was assumed that the two communicating sensors utilize signals from the sensor on each finger. Data were collected for about 5 minutes from each host at a sampling rate of 60 Hz. The ECG data for 10 subjects, on the other hand, were obtained from the PhysioBank database (`http://www.physionet.org/physiobank`). The ECG data were obtained from two leads on each subject. It was assumed that the two communicating sensors utilize signals from each lead for key agreement.

Performance analysis. Table 5.2 shows the parameters used in the feature-generation process. The basis for validation was satisfaction of the criteria discussed earlier in the chapter.

Table 5.2 PSKA feature-generation parameters

Signal	Parameters	Values
PPG	Sampling	60 Hz
	Sampling duration	12.8 s
	FFT	256 points, five windows[a]
ECG	Sampling	125 Hz
	Sampling duration	4 s
	FFT	256 points, two windows[b]
PPG/ECG	Peak-value quantization	5 bits
	Peak-index quantization	8 bits
	Feature length	13 bits

[a] The first 32 points per window were concatenated together for peak-based feature generation.
[b] The first 128 points per window were concatenated together for peak-based feature generation.

Long and random keys. The keys to be agreed upon are generated by the sender in the form of polynomial coefficients using a pseudo-random-number generator. The length and randomness of the keys agreed can therefore be ensured.

Low latency. The duration of sampling needed for secure key agreement varies according to the physiological signal and the technique used. With the PPG, which is sampled at 60 Hz, the best results were obtained with 12.8 s of data (due to the multiple-windowed FFT used to generate features); with the ECG, which was sampled at 125 Hz, this dropped to 4 s of data. In general it is observed that the more detailed the data available, the lower the latency.

Distinctiveness. An important requirement of PSKA is that the physiological signals can distinguish between people. This is important because the vault created by a sensor in one BAN must not be unlocked by another sensor located on another subject (either accidentally or maliciously) using features generated from its measurements. It is hence imperative to make sure that the number of common features for sensors on the same subject is "significantly" more than the number of common features for sensors on a different subject. The definition of significant is dependent upon the polynomial order v used. Figure 5.2 shows a graph of peak values versus peak index for PPG and ECG data obtained from the same individual and from different individuals. The lines which are completely superimposed are the common features. The higher the correlation between the FFTs of PPG and ECG signals at two sensors, the larger the number of peaks values and indexes they have in common in their respective FFTs. It can be seen from Figure 5.2 that sensors on the same person have a higher number of superimposed lines than do sensors on two different people. The lack of correlation between the FFTs of the physiological signals measured for two different subjects is due to the different physiological signature of each person at any given time.

Table 5.3 shows the statistics observed for the features when PSKA was executed with PPG and ECG signals. The difference between the number of common features for two sensors on the same subject and that for two sensors on two different subjects is significant. Therefore, given the statistic on differences in the number of common

Table 5.3 Benchmark Implementation: PPG/ECG feature statistics

Signal	Parameters	Values
PPG	Number of iterations	113, 1.6 s apart
	Average feature-vector length	~30
	Average number of common features (same host)	12
	Mode number of features (same host)	14.8
	Average number of common features (different hosts)	2
	Mode number of features (different hosts)	0.8
ECG	Number of iterations	180, 4 s apart
	Average feature-vector length	~87
	Average number of common features (same host)	24.7
	Mode number of features (same host)	25.2
	Average number of common features (different hosts)	9.5
	Mode number of features (different hosts)	8.1

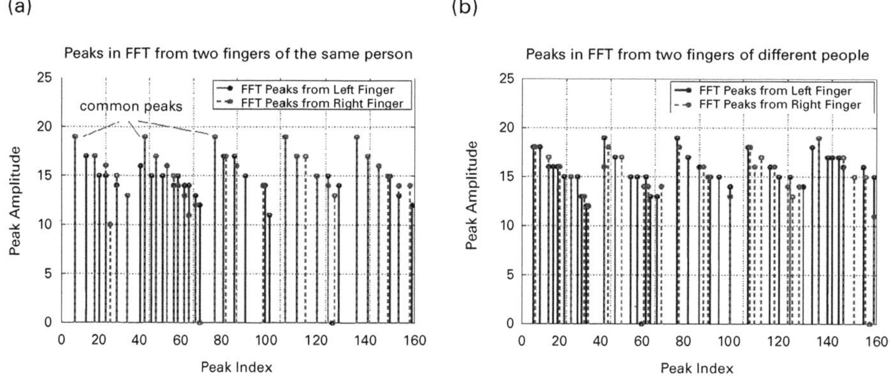

Figure 5.2   Benchmark implementation – PPG FFT peaks (peak index vs. peak values) for (a) the same host (total number of common peaks: 12) and (b) different hosts (total common peaks: 2).

features, the possible values for v can be derived. The polynomial order has to be such that the *false positives*, i.e., the number of times the common features between two people exceeds it, and the *false negatives*, i.e., the number of times the common features for the same subject is below it, are minimized. Figure 5.3 shows the percentages of false positives and false negatives when PPG and ECG data are used with PSKA for different orders of polynomials. For PPG data, the false-positive and false-negative rates are minimized when the order of polynomial used is 6, whereas for ECG data the optimal order of polynomial is 14. From these results it can be observed that using features derived from the PPG and ECG signals to generate a vault does not give any significant advantage to an adversary who uses features derived from another subject, provided that an appropriate polynomial order is chosen.

Temporal variance. Figures 5.4(a) and (b) show the temporal variance of the PPG and ECG signal features, respectively. The x-axis of the graph is the time difference

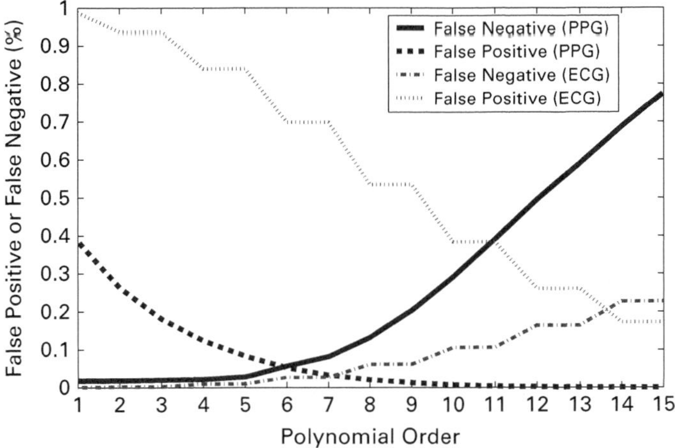

Figure 5.3   Benchmark implementation – false positive vs. false negative rate for ECG and PPG data.

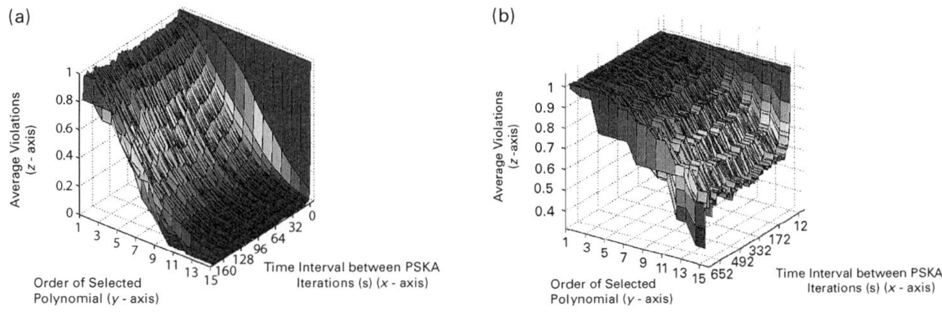

Figure 5.4   Benchmark implementation of temporal variance in (a) PPG features and (b) ECG features.

between the PPG and ECG measurement start times of two iterations of PSKA, the y-axis is the polynomial order used, and the z-axis shows the *average violation*, which is the percentage of times when the number of common features between the first and second iterations of PSKA is greater than the order of the polynomial used. As expected, when the time difference between the two iterations of PSKA both for the PPG and for the ECG is very close violations are very high, since the feature values in the two iterations are very similar. However, as the time difference increases the percentage of violations falls drastically for the PPG, reaching almost zero within the first few seconds for polynomials of order 9 and above. For the ECG with its higher number of common peaks between two different people, the fall in violations is more gradual and does not fall significantly before 14th-order polynomials and time difference of about 600 s between two PSKA iterations. Finally, as expected, both for the ECG and for the PPG, the higher the order of polynomial, the greater the number of common features needed and therefore the lower the chance of getting $v + 1$ common features between physiological-signal measurements at different time stamps.

Hence PSKA satisfies all the criteria set forth earlier in the chapter. The PPG-based PSKA requires a smaller polynomial order and shows more time variation than does the ECG-based PSKA. Interestingly, the plots of the temporal variation for the ECG and the PPG also illustrate the level of synchronization required between sensors when either is used as the physiological signal of choice. Both for the ECG and for the PPG the violations are highest when the time difference between the iterations is around 1 s, irrespective of the polynomial order used. This means that the features measured 1 s apart have not changed considerably, thereby still allowing successful unlocking of the vault. Therefore, even if the communicating sensors measure their physiological signals for PSKA 1 s apart (even longer for the ECG) they will succeed in agreeing on a common key.

Notice that these design goals of PSKA, if satisfied, can easily be shown to address the challenges associated with CPS-Sec (Section 5.2.2). The altered threat model of CPS is managed because of the private nature of the human body, which prevents easy tampering. The usability challenge is the principal one that PSKA as a CPS-Sec addresses, by allowing sensors to reach key agreement without any sort of intervention. The dynamic nature of the human body, in the form of topographic specificity, is compensated for by analyzing physiological signals in the frequency domain. Further, the dynamism of the physical process is utilized to enable improved security for the key-agreement process due to the time-varying nature of the features. Finally, in terms of computational and communication complexity there is a definite increase compared with manual key-distribution schemes. However, the footprint is low enough for one to execute about 8,000 iterations of PSKA on COTS sensors (Crossbow motes (`http://www.xbow.com`)) with two AA batteries [82]. Further, given the strength of the key exchanged as a result (which can be arbitrarily long), the process need not be repeated frequently, thus amortizing the cost.

5.5   Summary and future research problems

In summary, security is essential for BANs, given the sensitive nature of the data they collect and their actuation capabilities. Specifically, in this regard securing the communication between sensors is crucial. In this chapter, we focused on a new class of security solutions for securing BANs called CPS-Sec solutions. The idea is to use physical process features intimately with providing information security in a BAN context. This is achieved through PSKA, a scheme that utilizes the dynamic nature of the human body which produces chaotic, distinctive, and time-variant stimuli. The stimuli characterize the very specific situation the subject is in, and therefore make it difficult to predict current values even if past values are known. We presented a discussion on current techniques to achieve communication security with detailed analysis of a cyber-physical security scheme, PSKA, the issues involved in implementing it, its security capabilities, and performance results. This is by no means a solved problem. There are numerous issues that need to be handled.

The first is to redesign PSKA to make it more efficient and enhance its functionalities. Some of the possible avenues that can be investigated in this regard are (1) investigation of other (possibly simpler) physiological-signal-based features rather than FFT peak values and indexes for executing PSKA, which might have greater correlation and for which one need not use complex cryptographic primitives such as fuzzy vaults; (2) identification of newer physiological signals that exhibit lower topographic specificity; and (3) investigation of the use of physiological process models (human-body modeling) to determine the effectiveness of certain physiological signals in comparison with others for use with PSKA.

Further, at this point PSKA performs only pair-wise key agreement between sensors in a BAN. This may be sufficient for smaller networks, but, for managing very large networks, it is required to incorporate group-wise and network-wise key-agreement capability as well. An important line of enquiry could therefore be on extending PSKA to enable usable group and network key agreement with a minimal increase in the communication, computation, and memory overhead. The work on PSKA began with the goal of eliminating the need for communication during key agreement between sensors in a BAN by using synchronously measured physiological-signal features as keys. However, the topographic specificity of the physiological signals makes it very difficult to achieve this. One way to reduce the effects of topographic specificity is to use frequency-domain features. Therefore, it is worth investigating other signal-processing and cryptographic techniques, which can extend PSKA to perform key distribution without any form of communication exchange.

5.6 Questions

1. Why is security in BANs important? List the various aspects of the BAN which need securing. Why must they be secured?
2. An attack tree is a tree-like structure used to systematically study security issues in systems. Draw an attack tree for compromising BANs covering as many aspects as possible.
3. Create a taxonomy of the various types of adversaries that have the potential to attack communication in BANs.
4. Why is it essential to consider the environmental parameters in designing security solutions for BANs?
5. Can CPS-Sec solutions proposed for securing BAN communication be applied to secure the system against other than communication and actuation attacks in the attack tree? If so, which ones?
6. Why is time variation so important in PSKA? Why is not so important for biometrics? Can it be the other way around?
7. Think about ways of applying the concept of PSKA to other more realistic domains such as implantable medical devices (e.g., pacemakers and infusion pumps).
8. Can CPS-Sec solutions be used to secure a system against physical attacks on a BAN? If so, under what conditions? If not, why not?
9. Can CPS-Sec solutions aid in addressing availability (DoS) attacks on BANs? If so, in which context and why?

6   Sustainability

Environmental sustainability has been of increasing interest in designing any system in recent times. Computing systems usually contribute to this drive of sustainability from two different perspectives: (i) the energy perspective and (ii) the equipment-recycling perspective. Sections 6.1 and 6.2 describe these perspectives of sustainability of computing systems in general. All subsequent sections will focus on how to ensure sustainability for BANs from the energy perspective.

6.1   The energy perspective

Sustainability from the energy perspective, also referred to as energy-sustainability, has two main objectives: (i) reducing the carbon footprint from the power grid and (ii) reducing the need for battery replacement (for computing equipment running on limited-energy batteries). To ensure that both these objectives are attained, energy-sustainability can be described as the balance between the power required for computation and the power available from renewable or green energy sources (e.g., sources in the environment such as solar power). Ideally, if the power available from external renewable energy sources is more than the power required for computation then a power grid (or battery) might not be needed, and computation can be said to be energy-sustainable. However, in reality, both the available and the required power may vary over time. For example, solar power is available only during the day, but power may be required during the night (depending on the time-varying computing operations performed). In such a case, power may need to be extracted from a power grid (or battery) during the night, thus making computing operations unsustainable. In general, computing operations can become unsustainable when their power requirement is higher than the power available from green sources (as indicated in Figure 6.1). For energy-sustainability one thus needs to minimize the requirement for energy from the grid (or battery). Energy-sustainability can be generally defined as follows:

the energy-sustainability *is the average percentage of the energy used to power all computing units which is derived from green sources.*

However, there can be different manifestations of this definition. If there is no energy available from green sources (i.e., all of the computing operation has to be run from the grid or battery), then energy-sustainability boils down to reducing the average energy

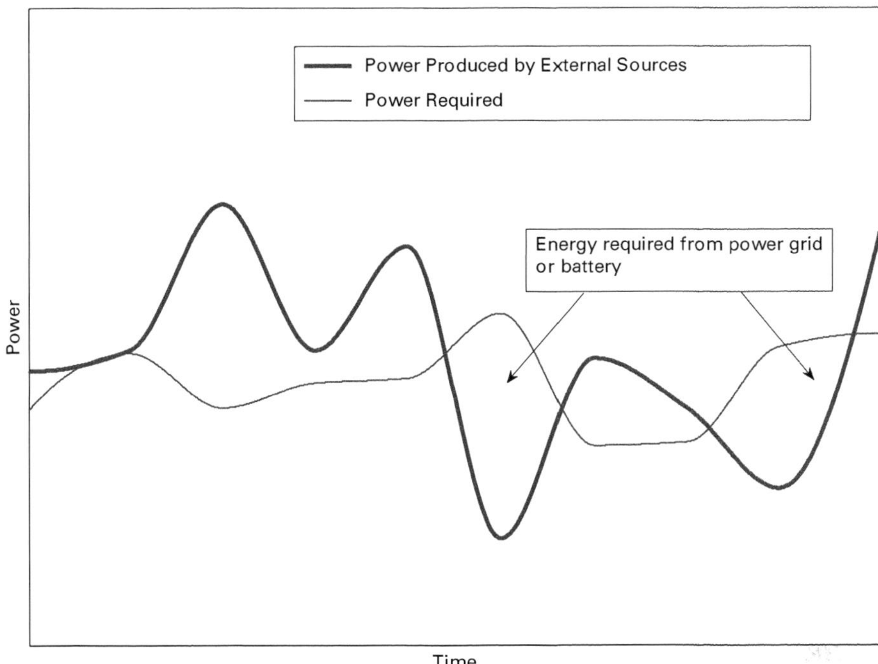

Figure 6.1 A profile of the power required and the power available from external (green) sources. Unsustainable operation can be caused by an imbalance of available and required power, in which case energy needs to be supplied from the power grid or battery.

required for the computing operations. Otherwise, energy-sustainability would require one to ensure that all computing operations are powered by energy generated from green sources as much as possible. In that case, *energy-sustainability can also be measured as the number of computing units that can be completely powered by energy from green sources*. Mechanisms to achieve energy-sustainability are described below.

6.1.1 Energy storage

Energy-storage devices can be used to store (and replenish) energy whenever energy is available from green sources. There have been several energy-storage techniques involving ultra-capacitors, compressed-air storage, batteries, fuel cells, and flywheels [123–125]. Figure 6.2 shows how unused energy (from green sources) can be stored (for the available and required power profiles in Figure 6.1). Unused energy can be accumulated in the storage device for later use. The stored energy can be used when the power requirement is higher than the power available from the green sources at any particular instant. The stored energy can later be replenished when the power required is less than the available energy from the green sources. Storage and replenishment of energy are ususally constrained by the energy capacity of the storage device, which imposes a limit on the amount of energy that can be stored. This limit may lead to situations in which energy produced by green sources cannot be used for later computations,

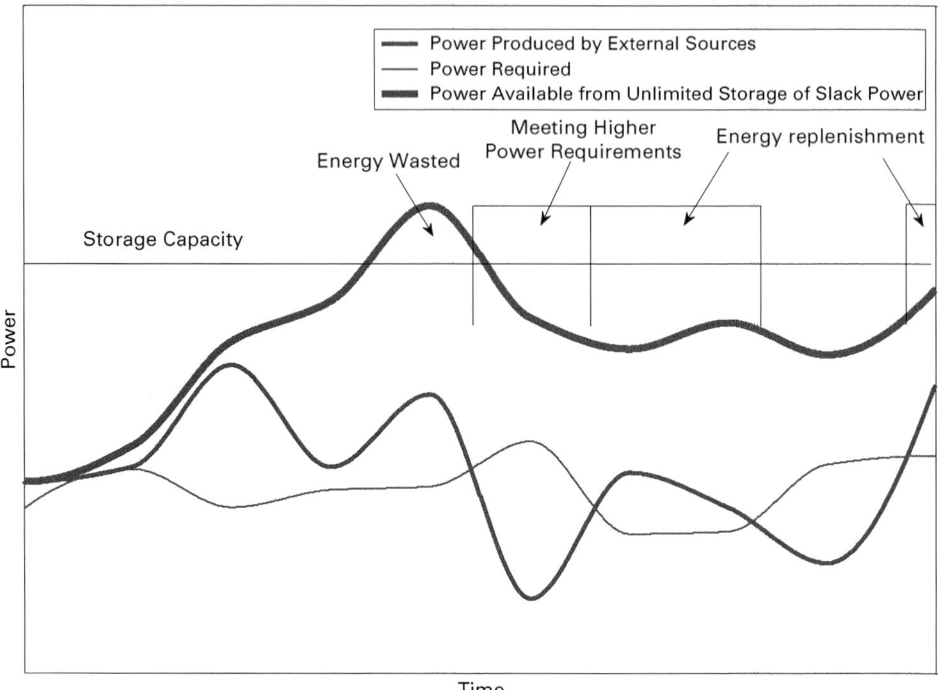

Figure 6.2   The power imbalance in Figure 6.1 can be addressed by storage of energy. At a given instant, the stored energy is the accumulation of the slack between the available and the required power for all the previous instants. Energy from the external sources can be wasted because of the limit on the storage capacity.

incurring wastage of energy (as shown in Figure 6.2). Such a situation can in turn lead to unsustainable operation if the power requirement is higher than the power available for long periods.

6.1.2   Reducing the energy requirement

Reducing the energy requirement can (i) allow one to completely avoid the afore-mentioned unsustainable operation by ensuring that the energy requirement becomes always less than the energy available from green sources (or a storage device) or (ii) reduce unsustainable operation by decreasing the need for energy from the power grid or battery. A reduction in the computing energy requirement is usually achieved in three ways.

1. *Spatio-temporal distribution of the computing operation.* Spatio-temporal distribution of the computing operation is widely known as workload (or job) management, and involves (i) ensuring that computing operations (jobs) are balanced across multiple computing units (as much as possible) in order to avoid overloading (and thus putting a high energy demand on) any single unit and (ii) delaying the

operations (within acceptable performance requirements) until power from green sources becomes available.

2. *Computing power management.* Another widely used method is to run the computing units in lower-power modes. For example, a processor not needed to perform any operation can be kept in *sleep* or *hibernate* mode to reduce the power requirement. Similarly, in a wireless network, radios can be turned on and off depending on the communication requirement (e.g., radio sleep scheduling in BANs [126, 127]). A survey on server-power and energy-management techniques has been published by Bianchini *et al.* [128].

3. *Non-computing system management.* The power requirement of the computing units is often supplemented by associated non-computing processes. Examples include energy requirements for cooling in modern data centers. Efficient management of the non-computing processes (e.g., cooling systems) can reduce the overall power requirement.

6.1.3 Scavenging energy from different sources

A complementary option (to reducing the energy requirement) for energy-sustainability is to increase the power available from one or more green sources. For BANs, Roundy *et al.* [129] and Paradiso and Starner [32] have provided a comprehensive list of means of energy scavenging from body heat, sunlight, ambulation, vibration, respiration, and so on.

This chapter primarily focuses on the energy-sustainability of BANs. Before that, the following section briefly touches upon sustainable computing from an equipment-recycling perspective.

6.2 The equipment-recycling perspective

Reusability and longevity of the computing equipment generally contributes to environmental sustainability by allowing recycling and decreasing the need for procurement, respectively. The mechanisms employed to ensure such sustainability are as follows.

1. **Ensuring failure-free operation.** Longevity of the computing equipment requires a high mean time before failure (MTBF), hence minimizing the requirement for replacing the equipment, especially since replacing sensors on the human body can be very cumbersome.

2. **Designing sustainable computing platforms.** Computing platforms can be developed using eco-friendly materials [130–132] to ensure that environmental sustainability can be maintained even with higher procurement of equipment.

6.3 Ensuring sustainability

Resources from the physical environment are used to extract green energy, which is used as the energy source in sustainable CPSes as discussed previously. However, associated with this mode of power supply are the problems of an intermittent energy source and unknown load characteristics. Moreover, the amount of energy available from the environment is often not sufficient to operate the computing units of CPSes. For example, it has recently been shown [32, 133] that the amount of power scavenged from the human body through body heat, ambulation, and respiration is not sufficient to operate state-of-the-art sensor operations at their maximum operating power. To overcome these problems, sustainability research has focused on three key techniques: (a) improving the efficiency of energy harvesting from the environment, (b) environment-aware duty cycling of computing units, and (c) energy-efficient computing.

Given these techniques, the goal of a sustainable design is to ensure that the CPS is *energy-neutral*. Energy-neutrality of a system essentially means that the system consumes as much energy as is harvested. Consider the SBCS power supply model in which at time $t = 0$ the battery capacity is $B(0)$. For energy-neutral operation of the system for δt onwards, the battery capacity at time $t + \delta t$ is also $B(0)$. In other words, the battery is never depleted for energy-neutral operation of a system. An analytic method for ensuring energy-neutrality of a CPS design has been presented in terms of the harvesting theory [134]. The harvesting theory takes a model-based approach, and considers stochastic models of the harvesting source and the computing unit. The harvesting source is modeled as a constant source of power ρ_1 with high- and low-standard-deviation margins of σ_1 and σ_2. The values of these parameters depend on the properties (**P**) of the physical environment, which is used as the scavenging source. The computing unit is modeled similarly as a constant power source ρ_2 with an upper limit of power consumption σ_3. The parameters ρ_2 and σ_3 will change for different energy-efficiency schemes employed to control the computing properties (**C**), such as the duty cycle and frequency. The energy obtained from the source is a function of ρ_1, σ_1, and σ_2, and can be considered as the interaction parameter.

The harvesting theory also models the inefficiencies of transferring energy from the scavenging source through the battery to the computing unit using a fraction η of useful energy and a parameter p_{leak} for leakage of energy. Given these models of the scavenging source, computing unit, and energy storage, the harvesting theory states that, for a system to be energy-neutral, the following criteria should be satisfied.

- $\rho_2 \leq \eta\rho_1 - p_{\text{leak}}$, which implies that on average the energy-efficiency technique should be such that the computing unit never consumes more power than is efficiently transferable from the battery.
- $B \geq \eta\sigma_1 + \eta\sigma_2 + \sigma_3$, which implies that the battery capacity B should always be greater than the maximum amount of power generated by the scavenging source plus the maximum power consumed by the computing unit. This criterion eliminates the possibility of energy wastage.
- $B_0 \geq \eta\sigma_2 + \sigma_3$, which implies that the initial battery level should contain the minimum level of power required to operate the computing unit.

Given this theoretical formulation of energy-neutrality, the harvesting theory can be used to design an environmentally aware duty-cycling scheme. The main observation in this regard is that all duty cycles are not equally essential. If the case of heart-rate measurement from PPG sensor data in a BAN is considered, the points of interest in the physiological signal are the peaks corresponding to a heart beat. The highest heart rate of a healthy human being never exceeds 200 beats per minute [135]. In such a case a duty cycle of more than 40% in an interval of 1 s is redundant, while a duty cycle of less than 30% causes loss of information. Hence, a utility function for the duty cycle can be defined, which assigns benefits to every possible duty cycle. The harvesting theory can then be used to find the most beneficial duty cycle of the computing unit in a CPS while maintaining energy-neutrality. In this regard, when one models the energy-scavenging unit it is essential to find the σ_1 and σ_2 parameters. To build these models, experimental characterization of properties of the physical environment, such as the diurnal variation of sunlight intensity and ambulation characteristics of the human subject, is necessary. Kansal *et al.* [134] discuss simple prediction methods for this purpose.

Thus, given some BAN hardware, the problem is that of how to develop for a given application the software which employs the available energy-management options to obtain a sustainable BAN, while meeting the computational requirements.

6.4   Sustainable BAN software-design methodology

Typically a BAN software-development process consists of three distinct phases that require information from the *physical plane*, which is the BAN system deployed on a human body, and the *management plane*, which consists of several management strategies as shown in Figure 6.3. The three phases of the software-design methodology (as shown in Figure 6.3) are (i) the profiling phase, (ii) the modeling phase, and (iii) the analysis-and-design phase.

In the profiling phase, experiments are performed on the BAN node to obtain workload-specific information regarding the processor, radio power, and thermal characteristics. Thus, in this phase the power consumption of the BAN node has to be evaluated for different power-management strategies under the application workload being considered. The node consists of both the processor and the radio, each of which has to be profiled. This phase includes also the profiling of scavenging sources to determine the amount of energy available from them throughout the scavenging period.

The data gathered from the profiling phase are then used in the modeling phase to build power models of the BAN. The main challenge in this step is to model the concurrent behavior of the BAN nodes and the human body.

The analysis-and-design phase consists of two interoperating subphases: (1) the analysis phase and (2) the design phase. The analysis phase takes a model and a set of requirements as inputs and outputs irrespective of whether the model properties satisfy the requirements or not. The design phase uses the analysis phase as a black box to work through the several design strategies and determine the optimal strategy for sustainable BAN design. The design phase iteratively reduces the search space by appropriately defining requirements and model inputs to the analysis phase, and achieves the optimal solution faster than would a brute-force search. The next sections describe the different planes and phases in the software-design methodology.

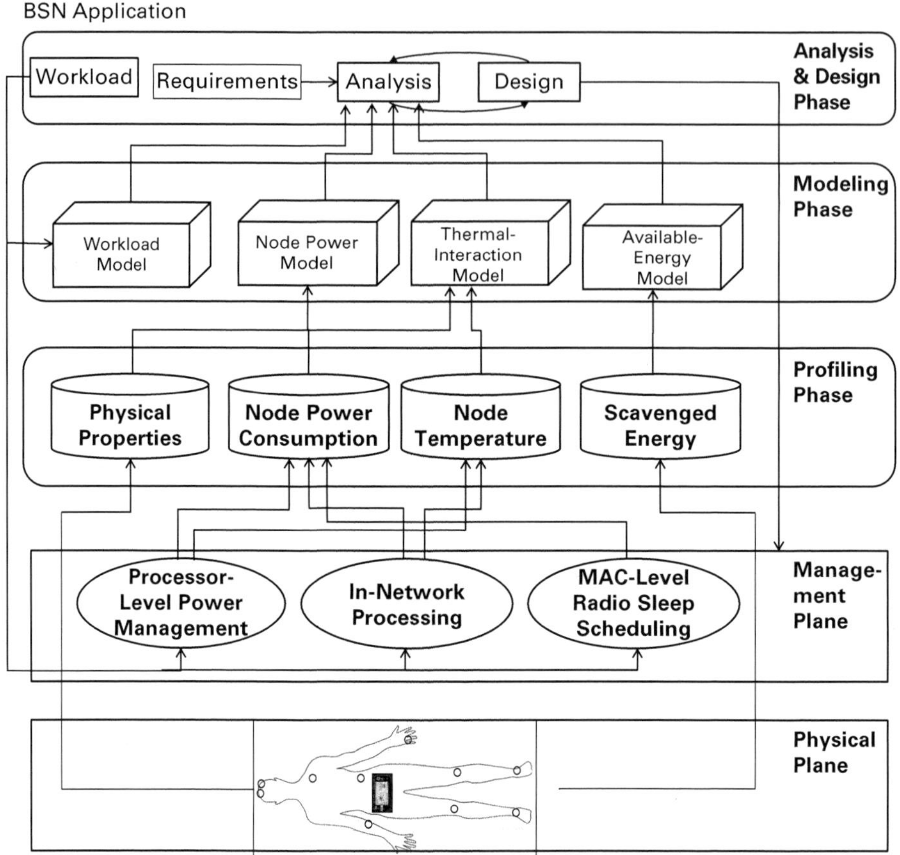

Figure 6.3   BAN software-design methodology.

6.4.1   The physical plane

A case-study is described in the following subsections as an example by means of which to discuss the physical plane in further detail.

The BAN hardware configuration

In this case-study, each BAN node consists of an Atom processor interfaced with a Chipcon radio (`www-inst.eecs.berkeley.edu/~cs150/Documents/CC2420.pdf`) for communication purposes. The Intel® Atom™ processor provides six sleep stages, of which the deep sleep state (C6) consumes the least amount of power. It also supports eight throttling modes in which the processor's operating frequency can be modulated. The sleep states and the throttling modes are controlled through an operating system called the Advanced Configuration and Power Interface (ACPI).

Scavenging nodes

In the literature [32], four sources for scavenging energy from the human body have been considered: (1) body heat, (2) respiration, (3) ambulation, and (4) sunlight. Paradiso and

Table 6.1 Available scavenging power

Scavenging source	Available power (W)	Scavenge time (h)
Body heat	0.1–0.15	24
Ambulation	1.5	2
Respiration	0.42	6
Sunlight	0.1	3

Starner [32] provide energy models of scavenging sources. Table 6.1 gives the available power from the scavenging sources and also the time durations for which they can perform the scavenging operation. The body heat and ambulation are the main sources of energy, given their high available power. Body heat is a continuous source of energy, allowing 24 h of scavenging operation. Any type of ambulation can provide a good amount of energy. However, ambulation might not be applicable for bedridden hosts. Scavenging from respiration can be used for a limited amount of time (6 h) since the scavenging process can impose respiratory strains on the host if used for longer. Sunlight is a limited source of scavenging energy, which can aid the main sources.

The human body

The mobility of a person may determine the amount of energy that can be scavenged. For example, energy scavenging from ambulation depends on the exercise pattern of the individual. Scavenging from sunlight depends on the frequency of outdoor visits by a person. Hence it is important to consider the mobility model while analyzing the effectiveness of a scavenging source.

Most researchers have used the random-way-point model as the mobility model for human users [67]. The random-way-point mobility model assumes that the probability of an individual moving to a point (x', y') from a point (x, y) is uniformly distributed. However, recent work has shown that the Lévy-walk model fits more accurately with the average human mobility pattern. The Lévy-walk mobility model assumes that the probability of an individual moving to a point (x', y') from (x, y) follows a Lévy distribution. This distribution can be skewed to match the tendency of an individual to prefer certain places over others.

6.4.2 BAN application

BANs are widely used in automated health care [136]. Hence, the Ayushman [54] privacy-enhanced health-monitoring application is considered as the computational workload. In Ayushman (as shown in Figure 6.4) the sensors in the BAN sense physiological data for t_s seconds and store them in local memory. After t_s seconds they transfer the data to the base station in a single burst. The data transmission can be performed using time-domain multiplexing, and is controlled by the MAC layer. Every communication is secured by encryption with a secret key, which is established for each pair of BAN nodes. Key agreement between two sensors is performed following the PSKA [137] protocol. In this protocol the two participating sensors sense the same

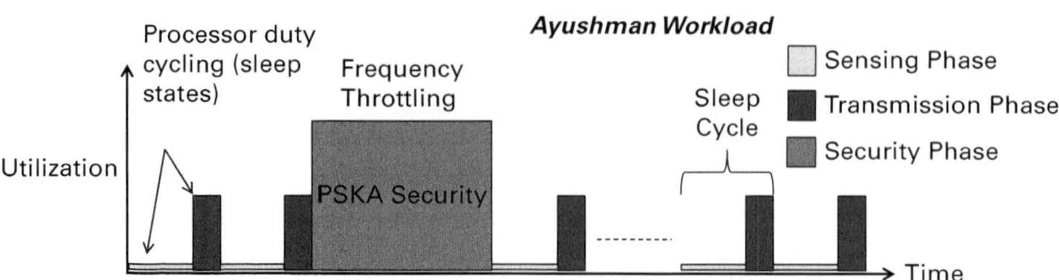

Figure 6.4   The BAN workload and application of design strategies.

physiological value (photoplethysmogram signals [137]), and perform complex signal processing, including FFT computation, peak detection, polynomial evaluation, and
quantization, to derive features. The features are used to hide a secret key using the
fuzzy-vault paradigm, and this key is exchanged between the two sensors (this process
is known as vault transfer). This secret key is used for further communications between
the two sensors. To maintain key freshness, PSKA execution is required every 24 h.

6.4.3   The management plane

The management plane consists of three main design strategies, which are employed to
achieve energy efficiency in BANs in order to ensure their sustainable operation.

1. Employing MAC-layer radio sleep-scheduling techniques.
2. Enabling processor duty cycling in individual BAN nodes.
3. Enabling processor frequency scaling in individual BAN nodes.

The application of the above-mentioned methods and their benefits in terms of energy-
efficiency largely depend on the workload characteristics as well as on the hardware
and software configuration of the BAN nodes. A typical BAN application, the Ayushman [54] health-monitoring application, as shown in Figure 6.4, is considered in the
case-study. It consists of intermittent high-activity computation and communication
phases followed by longer periods of inactivity. During periods of low computation
and communication, when the sensors are sensing data (Figure 6.4, short and wide
block), the processor can be put into a low-power sleep state and the radio can be shut
down. However, during data-transmission phases (Figure 6.4, tall and narrow block) the
processor and the radio have to operate simultaneously. In phases during which only
computation is required, as in the security phase (Figure 6.4, tall and wide block), the
radio can be shut down while the processor frequency can be modulated to control the
energy consumption.

6.5   Power profiling

Power measurements at the supply of the Mobile Intel 945 GSE (GMCH) chipset provide the board power consumption, which includes the CPU power as well as the power
for driving the chipset and other associated components. In order to isolate the CPU

Table 6.2 PSKA power usage

Operating mode (percentage throttling) (%)	Power consumption (W)
0	0.191
13	0.1864
25	0.17
37, 50, 62, 75	0.167
87	0.164

Table 6.3 PSKA execution time, RAM, and power consumption

Platform	RAM usage (%)	Power (mW)	Computation time (ms)
TelosB	80	66	2,186
Atom	0.006	164	41

power consumption during Ayushman execution, the idle power of the chipset can be measured for each throttling mode. The difference between the two power values gives the power consumed by the processor during the execution of PSKA, which is shown in Table 6.2 for different throttling modes. The resource and power consumption of Atom are compared with those of traditional BAN hardware (the TelosB mote). The power and RAM consumption of the PSKA algorithm in TelosB motes (using TinyOS) have been reported in [84]. Table 6.3 shows that the RAM consumption of Atom is far less than that of TelosB motes; however, even at the lowest operating frequency there is a threefold increase in power consumption. An interesting observation here is that the implementation of PSKA in TelosB motes [84] modified the algorithm and compromised accuracy, and hence the level of security, in order to keep the resource consumption within bounds. However, in Atom the implementation of PSKA is full-fledged, without any modification to the original algorithm [137]. Hence it provides a higher level of security while imposing a much lower RAM footprint. Further, even at the lowest operating frequency Atom has considerable speed up (by a factor of 50), and hence it does not violate the application's timing requirements.

The power consumption of the Chipcon radio was measured during transmission of packets at a bit rate of 250 kbps, which is standard for a sensor node (`http://www.xbow.com`). The current consumption of the CC2420 radio used in the BAN was measured to be 19.41 mA during reception and 19.20 mA during transmission. Considering the operating voltage to be 3 V, the maximum power consumption of the CC2420 radio is around 58 mW.

6.6 Architectural modeling

In this phase, the data from the profiling phase are used to develop functional models of the system in order to facilitate sustainability analysis. For a BAN the following components require modeling.

1. The BAN node. The essential properties of the hardware and software configuration are to be modeled for the BAN node. The properties which must be considered for sustainability are (1) the power consumption during execution of an application thread for different sleep states and operating frequencies, and (2) the core temperature of the BAN node processor.

2. Scavenging sources. The available amount of power from the scavenging source and the duration of scavenging are the important properties to be modeled.

3. Human mobility. Among several models of human mobility, the random way point, which is most commonly used, and the Lévy-walk model, which has been shown to fit the human mobility pattern the best, are considered.

Further, as shown in Figure 6.3, the modeling phase also requires a **workload model** for the BAN. The Ayushman application's workload is considered in this regard (Figure 6.4). The model building and specification can be performed using the industry-standard Advanced Architectural Description Language (AADL, www.aadl.info/). This is a hierarchical model-specification tool that provides constructs dedicated to modeling embedded software and hardware. However, it does not support modeling of the physical dynamics of the human body. Researchers have extended it [67] to incorporate specification of differential equations in the model to represent physical dynamics through the development of an annex (language extensions). The AADL specifications shown in this chapter denotes the AADL-specific constructs in bold.

The AADL Spec 1 gives the specification of the BAN system, which represents a BAN as a collection of subcomponents. The *BANnode.sensor* subcomponent implements the model of the sensor node (AADL Spec 4), *ScavengingSource.BodyHeat* models the scavenging source (AADL Spec 2), and the *HumanBody.skin* models the skin of the human body (AADL Spec 3). The BAN node is represented as a composition of three subcomponents: (1) a processor, (2) a radio, and (3) the application. The processor (*Processor.Atom*) power for different sleep states and the idle power consumption at various operating frequencies are obtained from the experiments performed during the profiling phase. The levels of busy power consumption of the processor for different operating frequencies are dependent on the application threads, and are modeled in the *Application.Ayushman* subcomponent.

AADL Spec 1 BAN-system specification

```
system implementation BAN.imp1
  subcomponents
  S1: system BANnode.sensor;
  B1: system ScavengingSource.BodyHeat;
  P1: system HumanBody.skin;
  connections
  C1: port ScavengingSource.BodyHeat → BANnode.sensor;
  C1: port BANnode.sensor → HumanBody.skin;
end BAN.imp1;
```

AADL Spec 2 Scavenging-source specification

```
system implementation ScavengingSource.BodyHeat
  properties
  AvailablePower => 100 mW;
  ScavengingTime => 24 h;
end ScavengingSource.BodyHeat;
```

AADL Spec 3 Human-body specification

```
system implementation HumanBody.skin
  properties
  SpecificHeat => 1.6 J/(kg.K);

     ...

  annex
  Del1<Temperature><Time> = K(Pdel2<Temperature><x>
+ Pdel2<Temperature><y> + Pdel2<Temperature><z>) + ...
end HumanBody.skin;
```

The model of the Ayushman application consists of three main threads: (1) sensing, (2) data transmission, and (3) PSKA execution, each of which models the power consumption and thread-execution time for a different frequency of operation of the processor. The *Radio.CC2420* subcomponent models the power consumption of the radio for three different modes of operation: (1) transmission, (2) reception, and (3) radio turned off.

The different models interact with each other to express the system's behavior. The interconnections of the models can be specified in AADL with the help of **ports** and I/O connections between them. As shown in AADL Spec 1 the power model of the scavenging sources interacts with that of the computing unit which is used in the sustainability analysis. The thermal data from the computing unit are transferred to the human-skin component for analyzing the temperature rise of the skin.

6.7 Analysis and design for sustainability

The analysis and design phase as discussed in Section 6.4 consists of two subphases: (1) design and (2) analysis. The design phase uses the analysis phase as a function, and calls it iteratively to reduce the search space for optimal design. The analysis phase obtains the requirements and the model of the BAN as input, and outputs whether the system meets the requirements.

Figure 6.5 shows a possible methodology employed to determine the optimal design strategy. Consider a set $M = \{m_1, m_2, \ldots, m_n\}$ of management strategies. For the case-study considered in this chapter, $M = \{F_1, F_2, \ldots, F_8, p, m\}$, where F_i is the ith frequency level of the processor, p indicates processor duty cycling, and m indicates MAC-level radio sleep scheduling. A design strategy is a combination of any number of management strategies. Thus, the set D of design strategies is a subset of the set 2^M

AADL Spec 4 BAN-node specification

```
system implementation BANnode.sensor
 subcomponents
 S1: system Processor.Atom;
 S2: system Radio.CC2420;
 A1: process Application.Ayushman;
    ...
end BANnode.sensor;

system implementation Processor.Atom
 modes
 SleepState1 : mode;
    ...
 Frequency1 : mode;
    ...
 properties
 IdlePower => 0.160 W in modes SleepState1;
 Temperature => 43 °C in modes Frequency1 ;
    ...
end Processor.Atom

system implementation Radio.CC2420
 modes
 RadioOnTx : mode;
 RadioOnRx : mode;
 RadioOnOff : mode;
 properties
 Power => 0.058 W in modes RadioOnTx;
    ...
end Radio.CC2420

process implementation Application.Ayushman
 subcomponents
 T1: thread Sensing;
 T2: thread PSKA;
 T2: thread Transmission;
end Application.Ayushman

thread implementation Sensing
 modes
 Frequency1 : mode;
    ...
 properties
 Power => 0.030 W in modes Frequency1;
 ExecutionTime => 5 s in modes Frequency1;
    ...
end Sensing
```

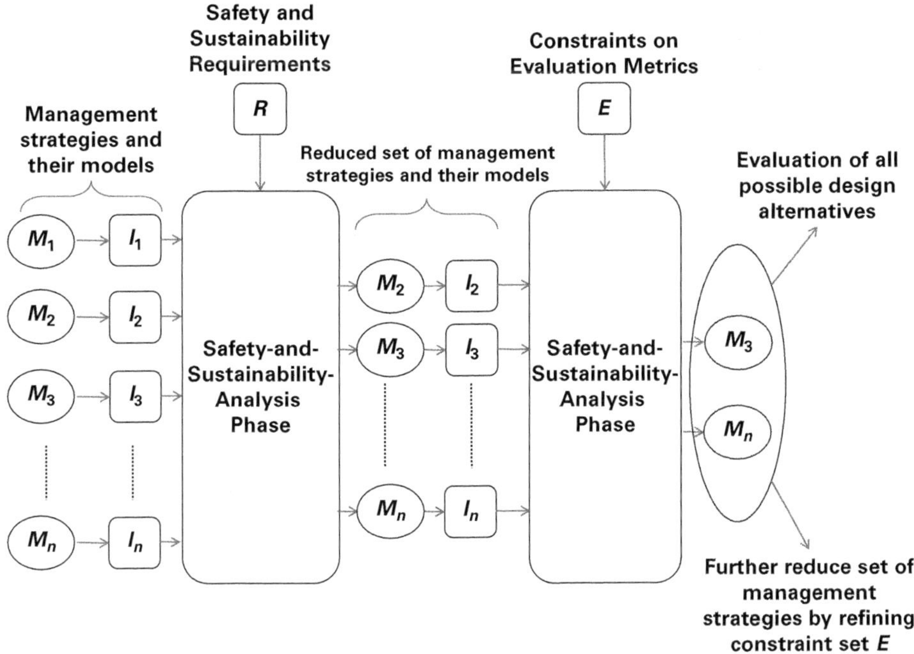

Figure 6.5   The design procedure.

(power set of M). Note that the set of design strategies may be a proper subset of 2^M if there are conflicts among the management strategies. For example, F_1, F_2 cannot be a management strategy since the processor cannot be in two frequency states at the same time. Further, let R be the set of sustainability requirements. Note that these requirements for sustainability can be a tuple (e.g., sustain 20 BAN nodes for 24 h of operation, denoted by the tuple $(20, 24)$). Each management strategy is then evaluated with respect to the requirements R using the sustainability analysis described in Section 6.7.1. For this purpose the model I_i for the management strategy m_i has to be fed to the analysis phase from the modeling phase (as shown in Figure 6.5). The analysis under the requirements R can be represented by the function $f_R : M \rightarrow M$. Since the management strategies in BAN are discrete in nature, failure to satisfy a requirement will eliminate the possibility of using that strategy. Thus, $f_R(M) \subseteq M$. In the next step design strategies d_i can be eliminated from the set D, which has a management strategy m_i such that $m_i \notin f_R(M)$. Let us call this reduced set D_R. It is intuitive that D_R is a subset of $2^{f_R(M)}$ since $f_R(M)$ are all the management strategies that remain. For the case-study, D_R is the set of subsets of the set $f_R(\{F_1, F_2, \ldots, F_8, p, m\}) = \{pF_8, mF_8\}$. This is because F_8, the lowest operating frequency for the processor, has already been fixed as a management strategy.

The next step in the design is to define evaluation metrics for evaluating the management strategies and further reducing the search space of the design. The evaluation metric is generally represented by a single value for a combination of system properties. For example, in the case of sustainability analysis the evaluation metric can be the number of BAN nodes sustained for 24 h of operation (**Number of sustained nodes**). For a particular BAN design, the developer would want to have certain specific values of the evaluation metric. For example, a designer might want to sustain 35 BAN nodes on the human body for 24 h of operation. This can be expressed as a set E of constraints on the evaluation metrics. Now the management strategies in $f_R(M)$ have to be evaluated using the analysis phase to determine the optimal design strategy (as shown in Figure 6.5). The execution of the analysis phase under the constraint set E is denoted by $f_E : M \rightarrow M$. Note that $f_E(f_R(M)) \subset f_R(M)$ such that any management strategy in $f_E(M)$ satisfies the constraints in E. The designer now has two choices: (1) perform a brute-force search on the reduced design phase $2^{f_E(f_R(M))}$ to find the optimal design, or (2) make a stricter constraint set E and repeat the analysis phase to further reduce the design space. The decision depends on the reduction in search space obtained due to the constraint set E. Given an initial state of management strategy M, the sustainability requirements constraint reduces the search space by a factor of $2^{n-|f_R(M)|}$. The employment of the evaluation strategy may further reduce the search space by a factor of $2^{|f_R(M)|-|f_E(f_R(M))|}$.

It is to be noted that the search space is still exponential. However, in the case of a BAN the number of management strategies is very low, for example 10 in this case, consisting of eight frequency levels, processor duty cycling, and MAC-level radio sleep scheduling. Thus, the search space in itself is small. Further, evaluating each design strategy with respect to sustainability requirements will require running the analysis phase described in Section 6.7.1 which is time consuming since it requires the solving of complex differential equations. Thus any reduction in search space can benefit the entire design procedure in terms of time requirements. The next section discusses the sustainability analysis under requirements R and constraints on the evaluation metrics E.

6.7.1   Sustainability analysis

The analysis phase takes the AADL model (I_i) obtained from the modeling plane and a set of requirements (R) as input. It first parses the model to generate a parse-tree representation of the AADL model, which is called **metadata**. From the metadata, model properties are obtained using APIs provided in the OSATE framework.

Algorithm 6.1 can be used for the sustainability analysis of a BAN design. The power consumption of hardware components (processor, radio) for execution of different threads (*Thread_Power*) and their timings (*Thread_Time*) are extracted from the AADL metadata. It is reasonable to assume that during the period of sensing t_s the Atom processor can be kept in C6 sleep mode, where it consumes P_{sleep} amount of power. For a BAN with n nodes the sensing process can be performed in parallel by all sensors. After each sensing period the sensed data are transferred to the base station. During this transmission period t_{Tx} the processor has to be in the active state, consuming P_{active} amount of power. The radio transmitter will also be active during this period (P_{radio} being its power consumption). Within a 24-h period there will be a number x of sense and transmit periods (wake-up cycles) for each sensor in the BAN, with a duration of $(t_s + t_{Tx})$

1: MetaData = ParseModel(AADL_BAN_Model)
2: [Thread_Power, Thread_Time, Scavenge_Power, Scavenge_Time] = ExtractProperty(Metadata)
3: NoOf_Required_wakeups = Calculate from Equation (6.2)
4: For each combination of scavenging technique
5:      Scavenge_Energy = $\sum$ *Scavenge_Power* × *Scavenge_Time*
6:      Sustained_wakeups = Calculate from Equation (6.3)
7:      while Sustained_wakeups > NoOf_Required_wakeups do
8:          Increase BAN nodes and repeat step 6

Algorithm 6.1 Sustainability analysis.

seconds each. Further, in a single day of operation of Ayushman the BAN nodes undergo pair-wise PSKA execution to maintain the freshness of the encryption key between two nodes. During this execution of PSKA the processor should be in its active state, consuming P_{PSKA} amount of power for the duration of execution of the PSKA algorithm t_{PSKA}. Further, during the transfer of the vault t_{Vault} the radio is active. Thus total energy consumption of the BAN is given by

$$\text{Total BAN energy} = \text{Sensing energy} + \text{Data-transmission energy}$$
$$+ \text{PSKA computation energy} + \text{vault-transfer energy}$$

$$\Rightarrow E_{BAN} = nx(t_s)P_{sleep} + nxt_{Tx}(P_{radio} + P_{active}) + t_{PSKA}P_{PSKA}\frac{n(n-1)}{2}$$
$$+ t_{Vault}(P_{active} + P_{radio})\frac{n(n-1)}{2}, \tag{6.1}$$

where x is determined from Equation (6.2), shown later. In a day there will be one pair-wise PSKA execution phase and x wake-up cycles. In a wake-up cycle it is assumed that the sensing is performed by all n nodes in parallel while the transmission of data is done in a TDMA fashion:

$$\text{Sensing time} + \text{transmission time} + \text{PSKA execution time} = 1 \text{ day}$$
$$\to (t_s x) + (t_{Tx})nx + (t_{PSKA} + t_{Vault})\frac{n(n-1)}{2} = 24 \times 3{,}600. \tag{6.2}$$

Table 6.4 gives the values of these variables, and also lists the methods for determining them. From the AADL model of the scavenging sources (*Scavenge_Power* and *Scavenge_Time*) the total scavenged and stored energy E_{TotSca} (*Scavenge_Energy*) is determined for each source (line 5 in Algorithm 6.1). During the PSKA execution and vault transfer, which happens only once in a day, the scavenging sources have to supply P_{PSKA} and $P_{radio} + P_{active}$ amount of power to the BAN nodes, respectively. The rest of the energy stored in the scavenging sources should sustain the operation of the BAN nodes for the rest of the day (i.e., provide enough energy to sustain x wake-up cycles).

Table 6.4 Parameter values

Parameter	Value	Methodology
t_s	5 s	Ayushman workload characteristics
t_{Tx}	0.39 s	Time taken to transfer 5 s of 32-bit data values sampled at a rate of 60 per second. The transfer rate is 24 kbps, which is standard for a Chipcon radio [84]
t_{PSKA}	0.0031 s	Measured time in Atom processor when running at 87% throttling
t_{Vault}	6.75 s	Calculated from the size of the vault and the Chipcon radio data rate [84]
P_{radio}	56 mW	Measurements from the Chipcon radio in TelosB motes [84]
P_{PSKA}	164 mW	Measured power of the Atom processor while executing PSKA at 87% throttling
P_{active}	160 mW	Idle power of the Atom processor [138]
P_{sleep}	80 mW	Power consumption of the Atom processor in C6 sleep mode [138]

The number of wake-up cycles, x_{sca} (*Sustained_wakeups* in line 6), that the scavenging source can sustain is determined from

$$x_{sca} = \frac{E_{TotSca} - (P_{active} + P_{radio})t_{Vault}n(n-1)/2 - P_{PSKA}t_{PSKA}}{(t_s P_{C6} + t_{Tx}(P_{radio} + P_{active}))n}. \tag{6.3}$$

If $x_{sca} > x$ then it can be concluded that the scavenging source can sustain the operation of the BAN throughout the day (line 7). Typically a single scavenging source is not enough to sustain the entire BAN. Hence, it is necessary to consider a combination of scavenging techniques in order to determine the maximum number of BAN nodes that they can sustain in a day. Evaluation metrics (E) can be defined, such as the number of sustained nodes, and the sustainability analysis can be represented by the symbol f_E.

6.7.2　Case-study design

In the first iteration of the design procedure, the top seven frequency states of the processor are eliminated since they do not satisfy the safety criteria. This is evident from Figure 6.6, which plots the **percentage of safety violation** for different frequency states. The reduced design space D_R now is a set of all subsets of the set of management strategies $M = \{p, m\}$. A brute-force search can be performed on this reduced design space, which gives us three possible cases:

(1) without any design strategy (NP–NM),
(2) with no processor-level power management but with MAC-level sleep scheduling (NP–M), and
(3) with processor-level power management and MAC-level radio sleep scheduling (P–M)

All the above-mentioned strategies consider operation at the lowest frequency. Given that the search space is small, an exhaustive search to determine the best possible solution, which maximizes the number of nodes sustained with minimum scavenging, is feasible. Figure 6.7 shows the number of BAN nodes sustained for 24 h of Ayushman

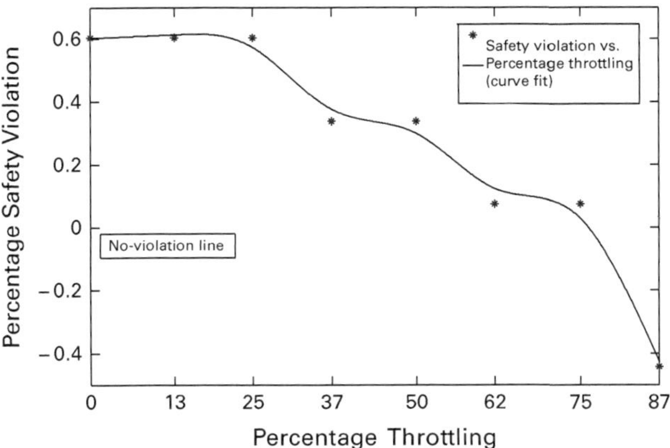

Figure 6.6 Safety-analysis results.

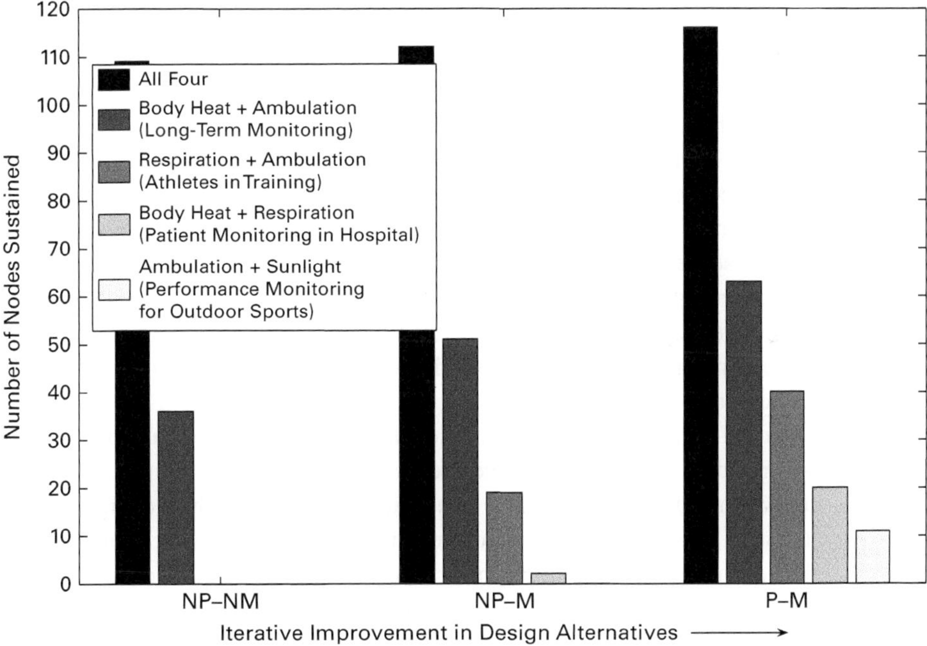

Figure 6.7 Sustainability-analysis results.

operation using the different scavenging combinations and for a particular design strategy. Combinations of scavenging sources are assumed according to their applicability in real-life situations. Scavenging from body heat and respiration can be applied for monitoring of bedridden patients in hospital. Ambulation and sunlight can be used in military applications or in performance monitoring in outdoor sports such as golf [139]. Ambulation and respiration can be used in the case of athletes in training. Body heat and ambulation can be used for long-term monitoring in a home environment. Figure 6.7

shows the number of BAN nodes sustained for each scavenging combination by arranging them in order of highest to lowest available scavenged energy. The absence of some bars from the figure indicates that the corresponding scavenging combination cannot sustain even a single node for 24 h. It can be observed that for the NP–NM strategy a sustainable design can be obtained if all four scavenging sources are used, or with a combination of body heat and ambulation. The P–M design strategy is the most efficient, sustaining up to 15 nodes with ambulation and sunlight (at the lowest available scavenged energy). These numbers will vary depending on the type and combination of scavenging sources, but the relative comparison of these strategies will remain the same. It is to be noted that an exhaustive search on all possible design strategies will require execution of the analysis phase 32 times. With the proposed design procedure the analysis phase is executed 11 times. Further, it has been observed by Banerjee *et al.* [67] that with context changes the time for which the nodes can be sustained decreases to 12.27 h on average, due to the intermittent nature of the energy availability.

6.8   Future research problems

One of the major unresolved problems in sustainability solutions concerns the efficiency of energy extraction from scavenging sources. The theoretical limit of the efficiency of a solar-electricity device is 70%, and it costs around $ 0.30 per kilowatt-hour (kWh) [140], an order of magnitude greater than current electricity costs. Further, the amount of energy scavenged per unit area of a source that extracts electrical power from the human body through body heat, respiration, or ambulation is very low [32]. Hence, to obtain the required amount of power, the form factor of the scavenger has to be increased. The development of a cost-effective and usable energy-scavenging source for CPSes remains to be done.

For effective environment-coupled duty cycling, scavenging sources have to be characterized in order to determine the maximum σ_1 and minimum σ_2 power generation. However, given the inherently intermittent behavior in their energy-generation characteristics, it is extremely hard to predict the amount of power available at a given time. For example, the amount of power available from a solar-electricity device depends on several environmental factors, such as the presence or absence of clouds and random obstructions providing shade. The characterization of the complex physical processes in the physical environment that affect scavenging and predicting the power available from a scavenging source at future time are open research problems.

The development of online predictive algorithms for the environment-coupled CPS workload is an important open problem. Being able to control the physical environment requires accurate characterization of the cyber-physical interactions during scheduling of the workload. Aperiodic arrival of workloads introduces uncertainties into such characterizations. Prediction algorithms for CPS workloads exist in different domains, such as for an Internet data center. They can be used to predict the behavior of the physical environment. However, the development of such prediction algorithms still remains an open research problem in application domains such as high-performance computing [141] and context-aware applications with sensor networks (`http://www.pranavmistry.com/projects/sixthsense/`).

6.9   Questions

1. What are the different perspectives of sustainability?
2. Why is the energy perspective important for BANs?
3. What is the power-imbalance problem?
4. Consider storage leakage in the battery. How would you modify Figure 6.2 to reflect storage leakage?
5. Consider the example of sensors on the human body being charged by scavenging sources through the wireless channel. Does this example need spatio-temporal modeling? If so, how would you use the GCPS discussed in Chapter 3 to model this example?
6. What is energy-neutrality? Why is it important?
7. Under what circumstances in Figure 6.2 can energy-neutral operation be guaranteed?
8. List the different sources of power dissipation in a BAN and compare their relative magnitudes.
9. What are the different strategies to reduce the computation power in a BAN?
10. What are the different strategies to reduce the communication power in a BAN?

7   Implementation of BANs

BANs are used in several smart and context-aware applications such as home-based health care [54], sports health management [142], entertainment [143], and military applications [144]. These applications impose several processing, communication, and storage requirements on the sensors in the BAN. For example, data sensing and storage are extensively required for home-based health care, computation-intensive physiological signal and image processing is required for military and entertainment applications, and online processing and communication of sensed data are used in sports health monitoring. Chapters 2 and 3 describe several BAN applications and their requirements in detail.

Usability issues in BAN, which include the need for easy wearability, infrequent re-charging of the battery, and thermally safe operation, prevent the use of powerful general-purpose processors in BAN sensors. Hence, application-specific developments of sensor platforms are essential for BANs. This has given rise to a plethora of sensor platforms that are being used for several BAN applications. These platforms are heterogeneous and typically limited in their computational, communication, and storage requirements. Processors ranging from powerful Intel xScale to low-power Atmega 128, radios ranging from power-hungry Bluetooth to efficient ZigBee, and storage ranging from 256 kB to 2 GB flash are available in current sensor platforms. Given these diversities in application requirements and sensor-platform capabilities, implementing a BAN application has two dimensions:

(1) choosing or designing a sensor platform that is best suited for a given application and
(2) implementing the given application in the sensor platform with stringent resource limitations.

This chapter discusses these implementation methodologies in detail. It discusses a systematic methodology by means of which to choose a platform that is most suited for a given application.

7.1   Implementation

We first look at the computation models of both the sensor and the base station.

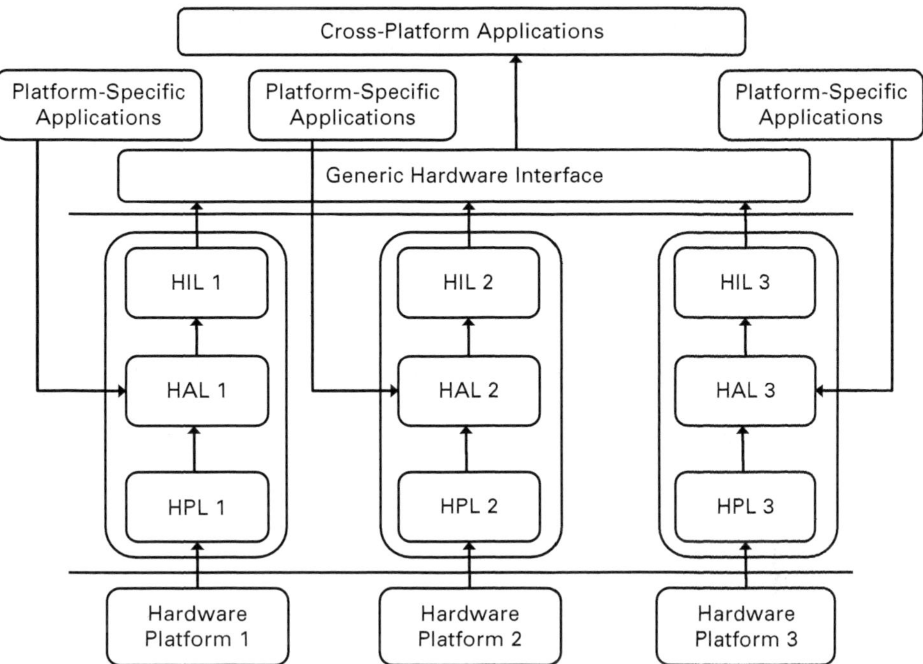

Figure 7.1 The TinyOS hardware abstraction hierarchy: HPL, Hardware Presentation Layer; HAL, Hardware Abstraction Layer; and HIL, Hardware Interface Layer. This figure has been derived from the figure in `http://www.tinyos.net/tinyos-2.x/doc/html/tep2.html`.

7.1.1 The computation model of a sensor node

The sensor-node computation model abstracts the underlying hardware using three layers as shown in Figure 7.1 (`http://www.tinyos.net/tinyos-2.x/doc/html/tep2.html`).

- The Hardware Presentation Layer (HPL). This layer directly communicates with the hardware interfaced with the sensor platform either through memory maps or by port-mapped I/O. The hardware generally communicates with the micro-controller by signaling an interrupt. The HPL handles these interrupts and provides five functionalities to the operating system for issuing commands and obtaining responses from the hardware:
  - *start* and *stop* commands for the powering up and down of the hardware device,
  - *get* and *set* commands to read and write the registers associated with the hardware,
  - commands for enabling and disabling interrupts generated by the hardware,
  - service routines for the interrupts, which are often called *event handlers*, and
  - customized functions for operating on flags specific to a given hardware component.

  Each item of hardware interfaced to the sensor platform has these three layers of abstractions, which represent the hardware as a black box with *interfaces*, namely inputs and outputs, *events*, namely actions undertaken during asynchronous occurrences of events, *tasks* that can be used to post the execution of certain functionalities for a later time, and *functions*, which are used to execute a piece of code immediately.

- The Hardware Adaptation Layer (HAL). This layer of abstraction lies above the HPL, which further abstracts the basic interfaces provided by the HPL for hardware to task specific interfaces. For example, if two sensors provide the same universal asynchronous receiver/transmitter (UART) interface then the HAL groups them into one. The application can distinguish between the two sensors by properly wiring the UART interface to the appropriate HPL components.
- The Hardware Interface Layer (HIL). This a higher level of abstraction than the HAL. It takes the interfaces provided by the HAL and represents them as application-specific functionalities. For example, a HIL can take a sensor and timer component and build a new component that allows an interface to periodically query the sensor.

TinyOS (`http://wwww.tinyos.net`) is an operating system designed specifically for wireless sensor networking. It has a simple first-in, first-out (FIFO) scheduler that schedules threads and supports multi-threading. TinyOS has two types of threads.

- *Task threads.* These threads are used for long-running computation-intensive operations. Tasks can be posted for execution at a later time. Whenever a task is posted, it is registered in the FIFO queue of the scheduler and is executed whenever the microcontroller is free. Tasks are non-atomic and can be halted by asynchronous interrupts or other tasks occurring in parallel.
- *Event threads.* These are asynchronous interrupts associated with events occurring in hardware such as a packet being received by the radio or a request for direct memory access (DMA) being made by sensor hardware. Event threads are used for short-running operations such as setting a variable, posting a task, or firing a timer. Event threads are atomic and cannot be interrupted.

7.1.2 The computation model of a base station

In this chapter, we consider a mobile phone as the base station and discuss the computation model of Android (`http://www.android.com`), a Linux-based operating system for smart phones.

Android is a software stack running on top of a Linux kernel; hence it uses the Linux paradigms for scheduling threads and multi-tasking. It provides four constructs to an application, which the application can use to execute complex operations, access services from different components of the base-station hardware, communicate with other applications, and manage content in a systematic way. These constructs are as follows.

- *Activity.* Each application extends an activity in Android. An activity is the equivalent of a thread in the Linux operating system. The activity uses objects and functions to execute complex operations. They can interact with the user and request data or services from other activities or services via queries or intents (which will be discussed later).
- *Services.* Each hardware component in the base-station device extends a service to the Android software stack. For example, the Bluetooth radio will extend a

communication service to the Android software stack that can be accessed by any running activity. The services continue to run in the background and provide interfaces to the activities until the base station is shut down.

- *Broadcast and intent receivers.* These are interfaces used by activities to communicate with services. A broadcast receiver is a system-wide event or interrupt indicating events in a service. For example, a packet being received by the Bluetooth module is an event that can be registered by the broadcast receiver. Intent receivers are used to create new activities from existing ones. These enable an activity to select another activity on the basis of the actions to invoke and the data to operate on. Data can be passed in both directions using intent objects, and this enables a convenient, high-level method for inter-process communication.
- *Content providers.* These are interfaces used for accessing information from services and activities in a standard format.

7.2 Programming paradigms

The programming paradigms of a sensor and of the base station are very different. The base station has an imperative programming model whereby it follows a definite sequence of steps in an algorithm. However, the sensor's programming paradigm is event-driven, whereby the sequence of execution is random and determined by events detected by the sensor. The following sections demonstrate the programming of a TinyOS-based sensor with an Android mobile phone as the base station.

7.2.1 Programming a sensor

In TinyOS a sensor-side application has two parts. The first part, the *module*, instantiates different hardware abstractions for use in the application and writes the functions, event handlers, and tasks, while the second, the *configuration*, wires the abstractions to the desired hardware components.

We discuss these two parts in detail with the help of Example 7.1.

Example 7.1. *Consider a sensor application, where the sensor platform uses the light sensor and then transmits the light intensity value to the base station through the Zig-Bee radio. The module part of the code first instantiates the interfaces of the hardware abstractions. As shown in the code segment Algorithm 7.1, the sensor uses the Boot interface to boot up, Receive, AMSend, Packet, and SplitControl interfaces to control the ZigBee radio, and the Read interface to read from the sensor. As can be seen from the code segment, one can rename the interfaces with specific semantically meaningful names.*

For each hardware component instantiated, all of its function and event handlers have to be implemented in the implementation *section of the module. As shown in the code segment Algorithm 7.2, all of the events for the RadioControl interface have been implemented.*

```
module RadioSenseToLedsC {
  uses {
    interface Boot;
    interface Receive;
    interface AMSend;
    interface Packet;
    interface Read<uint16_t>;
    interface SplitControl as RadioControl;
  }
}
```

Algorithm 7.1 Interface declaration in TinyOS.

The configuration part of the code in the sensor instantiates hardware components in any of the three abstraction levels listed in Section 7.1.1. It then wires the interfaces instantiated in the module section to the hardware components instantiated in the configuration section of the code as shown in the code section Algorithm 7.3.

7.2.2   Programming a base station

The base station is programmed using the Android software stack. The Android software stack is implemented in Java and provides several system-specific plug-ins and classes to access the different functionalities of the base-station device, which is typically a phone. The Android software has dedicated classes for the creating a graphical user interface (GUI) in the phone. Each GUI class has events associated with it, such as button press, click, or highlight. Complex algorithms can be implemented in these event handlers using the Java programming paradigm. In the code sample Algorithm 7.4 we show the display of text on the phone screen.

Here the TextView class is used to create a text box on the phone screen. The onCreate event is fired whenever the application is started. In the onCreate event handler the TextView class is instantiated as an object. Its setText function is then used to write the "Hello, Android" text on the screen.

Apart from simple GUI classes the Android software stack also provides classes to access services such as the Bluetooth receiver, intent-receiver classes to communicate with other applications, and content-manager classes to handle data.

7.3   Common implementation issues

Implementing applications in sensor platforms is challenging due to their resource-constrained nature, slow processing capability, and real-time processing requirements. In this section, we list some common implementation issues and provide some "tricks" by means of which to overcome them.

```
implementation {
event void RadioControl.startDone(error_t err) {
  call Read.read();
}
  event void RadioControl.stopDone(error_t err) {}

  event void Read.readDone(error_t result, uint16_t data) {
    if (locked) {
      return;
    }
    else {
      radio_sense_msg_t* rsm;
      rsm = (radio_sense_msg_t*)call Packet.getPayload(&packet, NULL);
      if (call Packet.maxPayloadLength() < sizeof(radio_sense_msg_t)) {
return;
      }
      rsm->error = result;
      rsm->data = data;
      if (call AMSend.send(AM_BROADCAST_ADDR, &packet,
sizeof(radio_sense_msg_t)) == SUCCESS) {
locked = TRUE;
      }
    }
}

    event message_t* Receive.receive(message_t* bufPtr,
     void* payload, uint8_t len) {
      call Leds.led1Toggle();
      if (len != sizeof(radio_sense_msg_t)) {return bufPtr;}
      else {
        radio_sense_msg_t* rsm = (radio_sense_msg_t*)payload;
        uint16_t val = rsm->data;
        return bufPtr;
      }
    }

    event void AMSend.sendDone(message_t* bufPtr, error_t error) {
      if (&packet == bufPtr) {
        locked = FALSE;
      }
    }
}
```

Algorithm 7.2 Implementation of sample sensing and sending through ZigBee in TinyOS.

7.3.1 Avoid floating-point operations

Floating-point operations in a sensor require complex processing and are very slow compared with fixed-point operations. Often it is beneficial to represent floating-point

```
configuration RadioSenseToLedsAppC {}
implementation {

// Component declaration

  components MainC, RadioSenseToLedsC as App, new DemoSensorC();
  components ActiveMessageC;
  components new AMSenderC(AM_RADIO_SENSE_MSG);
  components new AMReceiverC(AM_RADIO_SENSE_MSG);


// Wiring

  App.Boot -> MainC.Boot;

  App.Receive -> AMReceiverC;
  App.AMSend -> AMSenderC;
  App.RadioControl -> ActiveMessageC;
  App.Packet -> AMSenderC;
  App.Read -> DemoSensorC;
}
```

Algorithm 7.3 The configuration section of a TinyOS code with components instantiated in the declaration part and wired to the abstractions declared in the main code.

```
package com.example.helloandroid;
import android.app.Activity;
import android.os.Bundle;
import android.widget.TextView;
public class HelloAndroid extends Activity {
  /** Called when the activity is first created. */
  @Override
  public void onCreate(Bundle savedInstanceState) {
      super.onCreate(savedInstanceState);
      TextView tv = new TextView(this);
      tv.setText("Hello, Android");
      setContentView(tv);
  }
  }
```

Algorithm 7.4 The Android "Hello World" program.

numbers in fixed-point format and use fixed-point arithmetic on them. This also helps in reduction of memory usage since floating-point numbers are usually represented using 32 bits. However, most of the sensor applications will not require such high resolution. Hence, in such cases floating-point numbers can be represented using 16-bit fixed-point numbers. One such example representation is to use a three-step process as follows. (1) The floating-point numbers are represented in binary-point format. (2) The binary-point representation is shifted seven places to the right and all the bits to the right of the binary point are ignored. (3) The bits to the left of the binary point are then used to represent the floating-point number in the 32-bit fixed-point representation. The principal idea behind the process is to multiply the floating-point number by 128 and store the integer portion of the result. This effectively provides a representation of the floating-point number with a precision of two decimal places. Given the fixed-point representation of floating-point numbers, a framework for basic arithmetic operations on floating-point numbers such as 32-bit floating-point addition, subtraction, multiplication, division, comparison, and exponentiation can be developed. However, there are two basic problems with such a representation.

- There are inaccuracies in the representation of the decimal part of the floating-point numbers. Such inaccuracies can get amplified due to a wrong order of execution of arithmetic functions. For example, consider division of 0.3 by 5 and multiplying it by 20, whose answer should be 1.2. If we consider doing the division first and then the multiplication, we would get 140 as the answer, which is the fixed-point representation of 1.09. This is due to the truncation of the decimal part in the division step. However, if we consider multiplication first and then division, then we get an answer of 153, which is the fixed-point equivalent of 1.19. Hence, the inaccuracy depends on the sequence of execution of the functions.
- Even if the individual numbers and the results of arithmetic operations on them do not require a 32-bit representation, integer overflows may happen in intermediate steps when all numbers are represented as 16-bit fixed points. For example, in the case of performing a multiplication operation on two numbers and then division, even if the result is in 16 bits, the multiplication operation can cause integer overflows. Hence, the strategy of representing floating-point numbers as 16-bit fixed-point numbers for memory management has to be carefully pursued.

7.3.2 Variable reuse and concurrency conflicts

Variable reuse, although a bad practice in software development, is one of the common strategies used for reduction in memory usage in sensors. However, given the concurrent-execution model of TinyOS, such strategies can cause serious problems. For example, consider a global variable that is reused in two tasks. If the tasks are executed in parallel then the same variable can be updated at two different places, and the execution will give erroneous results. To practice variable reuse in a concurrent-execution environment complete isolation of the tasks is required, ensuring that when one task is executing the other task using the same variables has not yet been posted.

7.3.3 Storage management

There are two types of storage in a sensor: (a) RAM and (b) flash memory. The RAM is typically very limited in size, typically 10 kB for commercially available sensor platforms, while the flash memory is orders of magnitude higher in size (nearly 2 GB). However, the access latency for RAM is significantly lower than that of flash memory. Hence, intelligent storage management is required in order to optimize performance and memory-resource usage. Typically, the buffers used to store sensed signals, or coefficients of FFT processing, which are used rarely, are not likely to change, and can reach huge sizes, are kept in flash memory. However, variables that are used frequently in the program execution are kept in the RAM.

7.3.4 Distinction between tasks and event handlers

Event handlers are used for fast and simple processing, whereas tasks are used for more complex and time-consuming processing operations. Hence it is important to limit the computation in an event handler solely to flag settings and timer initiations. As an example, consider that a timer is being fired at repeated intervals and a radio receive is registered in parallel. In such a scenario, if in the radio-receive event handler the program takes a long time to execute then the timer fire event may occur during the program execution. However, events are atomic operations, and cannot be interrupted. Hence, the timer-fired event may be ignored in such a scenario. If a complex time-consuming operation is to be performed, it can be posted as a task and placed in the scheduler FIFO queue for concurrent execution.

7.3.5 Real-time considerations

Consider the example in Section 2.3, where ECG signals are sensed and time-consuming operations such as peak detection, FFT computation, and signal-correlation computation are performed. A 2-s sample of ECG signals is stored in a buffer on which these operations are performed. If we follow a sequential approach to computation, then we first store the data in a buffer, stop sensing and perform only computation on the stored signal, and then again start sensing. In this approach, a significant portion of the ECG time series is lost when the sensor node just processes and does not sense. To make it a real-time operation, two buffers (A and B) are required. When processing is done on the stored signal in buffer A, the sensing can occur in parallel and store sensed values in buffer B. Then the processing can switch to buffer B while sensed values are stored in buffer A. However, the size of the buffers A and B depends on the time taken to process the stored signal in the buffers. If the processing takes a long time then a large amount of data will have to be stored. For example, the processing for the application shown in Section 2.3 takes approximately 4 s to execute. To prevent any loss of data there a buffer needs to store 600 samples of ECG data at a sampling frequency of 125 Hz, which means an extra storage of 1.2 kB. However, since computation on this 4 s of data will be performed at a later time, it can be stored in the flash memory rather than in the RAM. Hence, with intelligent use of storage real-time operation of the sensor can be achieved. Such considerations are extremely important during implementation in an embedded platform.

7.3.6 Debugging strategies

Debugging embedded platforms such as sensors is problematic due to the lack of sophisticated runtime error detectors. Sensor nodes do not have any error-reporting scheme such as those available for high-level programming languages such as Java and C. Hence, when an error occurs in a sensor node, it is extremely difficult to trace back the source of the error. There are three possible methods by which to debug a sensor-node code.

1. Use of emulators. TinyOS provides an emulator called Tossim that can be used to test the execution sequence of a sensor-side code. It can be used to detect errors such as segmentation faults, infinite loops, and array overflows. However, Tossim is very much limited to the micaZ platforms developed by xbow and does not support the use of platform-specific components for other devices such as TelosB and Shimmer.
2. Use of on-board LEDs. On-board LEDs can be used to see whether the execution sequence is as expected. These LEDs can be toggled or turned on in a function or event handler to check whether the execution goes through that piece of code.
3. Communicating with the base station. Variables of interest can be communicated back to a desktop base station where they may be compared with the desired value to check correctness of the operation. In this regard, a MATLAB-based base station is often useful to visualize the variables in the sensors.

7.4 Diverse sensor platforms

Sensor platforms typically consist of a micro-controller, a radio, an antenna, external memory, and other peripheral components integrated on a single circuit board. Several platforms such as Shimmer [145], Tempo 3.1 [146], BSN node v3 [147], TelosB [148], and iMote2 [149] are used for experimental deployments and clinical trials in BAN research. There exists a significant variety among these platforms in terms of components, form factor, and overall design. For example, the iMote2 platform has a separate coprocessor for signal processing, while other platforms use a single microprocessor. The TelosB platform uses an inverted-F antenna, Shimmer uses a chip antenna, and iMote2 uses a surface-mounted antenna. Many custom-made sensors use field-programmable gate arrays (FPGAs) for fast hardware implementations of specific functionalities such as FFT computation. In an FPGA, the interconnects and logical blocks can be used to develop any digital system. Further, they have re-configuration capabilities, whereby the hardware can dynamically adapt to serve different logical functionalities. Recent advances in the development of embedded systems have led to the design of Intel's TunnelCreek platform, which interfaces the Intel Atom processor with ASICs and FPGAs. In such a scenario, an application can be divided into functional blocks, and different blocks can be intelligently implemented in different hardware resources to achieve speed and energy-efficiency.

7.5   Choosing the best platform

Given the diverse nature of BAN applications and the diverse capabilities of platforms available for BANs, it is important to choose the correct platform that has the right set of capabilities for the given application. In this regard, an application-driven platform-evaluation framework is of extreme importance. We describe here the evaluation framework described in [150]. This evaluation framework is composed of two phases: design-space determination and design-space exploration, as shown in Figure 7.2. The design-space determination phase starts by identifying a set of salient features of a BAN platform that determine its performance in BAN applications. These need not necessarily be individual physical components of the platform (e.g., a microcontroller or radio), but instead are specific aspects of the platform's performance (e.g., communication reliability, processor performance) that influence its suitability to a given BAN application. These features are considered as *design coordinates*, and are used as a common basis for comparing a diverse set of platforms. The multi-dimensional space defined by these coordinates is referred to as the *design space*. The next step is to quantify these coordinates using suitable metrics. These metrics are based on an application-oriented view of each coordinate. That is, for each design coordinate, we investigate how it affects the performance of the overall platform in a BAN application, and provide a quantitative measure of this effect.

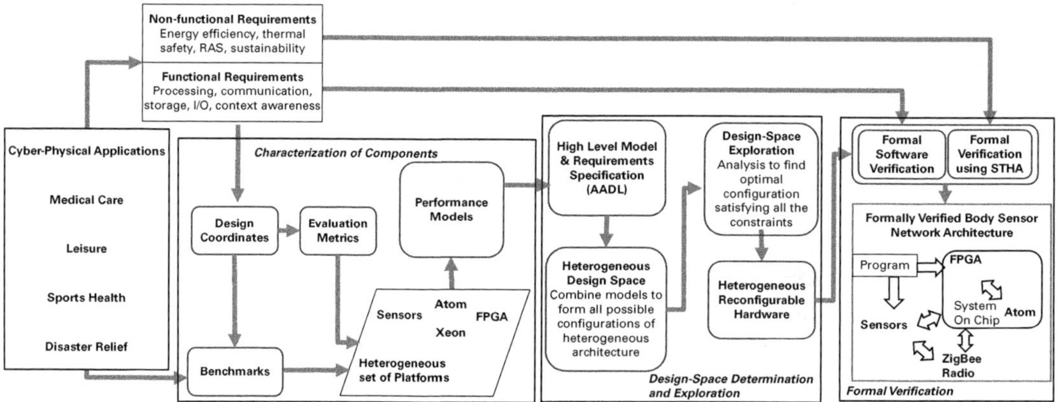

Figure 7.2   A two-phase evaluation framework: design-space determination and design-space exploration. The design coordinates defining the design space are chosen on the basis of the platform requirements of typical BAN applications.

Once the set of design coordinates and the corresponding metrics have been identified, the next step is to evaluate a platform derived from these metrics. This must be done under typical BAN application workloads in order to obtain a realistic, practical characterization of the platform. This can be accomplished by using a BAN-specific benchmarking suite such as *BSNBench* (`http://www.ee.washington.edu/research/nsl/BSNBench/downloads.html`). BSNBench is based on the observation that BAN applications, despite their being highly diverse, have some basic tasks that are common to all of them. BSNBench is composed of such basic tasks, and each task focuses on evaluating a single design coordinate. Having obtained a numerical value for the coordinates of a platform, each platform can be mapped to a point in the design space.

In the design-space-exploration phase, a set of application requirements is mapped to the platform design space in the form of *constraints* to define a suitable subspace. A platform lying within this subspace is considered suitable for the given application. Further, for platforms lying outside the desired subspace, their distance from the subspace indicates the need for improvement in their design. This distance can be decomposed along individual design coordinates to identify specific components of a platform that must be improved in order to make it suitable for the application. For the design of new BAN platforms, the design goals are expressed as objective functions of the design coordinates, and are evaluated over the desired subspace in order to identify the optimal design point.

7.6 Automatic code generation

To implement an application in the smart phone and the sensor, a developer must be proficient with the operating system and hardware of the embedded devices. Further, ensuring that the implementation of the BAN will satisfy the requirements set forth in the model-based-analysis phase requires optimized implementations. Manual implementation of these models may introduce errors, which may in turn lead to requirements being violated by the BAN implementation. In this regard, researchers have proposed automated implementation of BAN from their models.

Recent research has concentrated on developing APIs for TinyOS-specific sensor-code generation. There exist several works on API development for TinyOS to support signal processing, intelligent storage, and energy-efficient communication [151–153]. However, to use these APIs the user has to write TinyOS code for the sensors, introducing the possibility of errors. The mobile middleware [151] provides a basic API for the smart phone to control the sensors.

Researchers have also focused on code generation for sensors from a high-level specification such as Simulink [153], or graphical specifications [154–156]. The framework proposed in [153] can generate code for TinyOS-based sensors, and also supports algorithm-execution sequences. RaPTEX [154], Viptos [155], and TOSDev [156] consider the sensor nodes as some of the tools used to automatically generate TinyOS-based sensor code from high-level models and specifications.

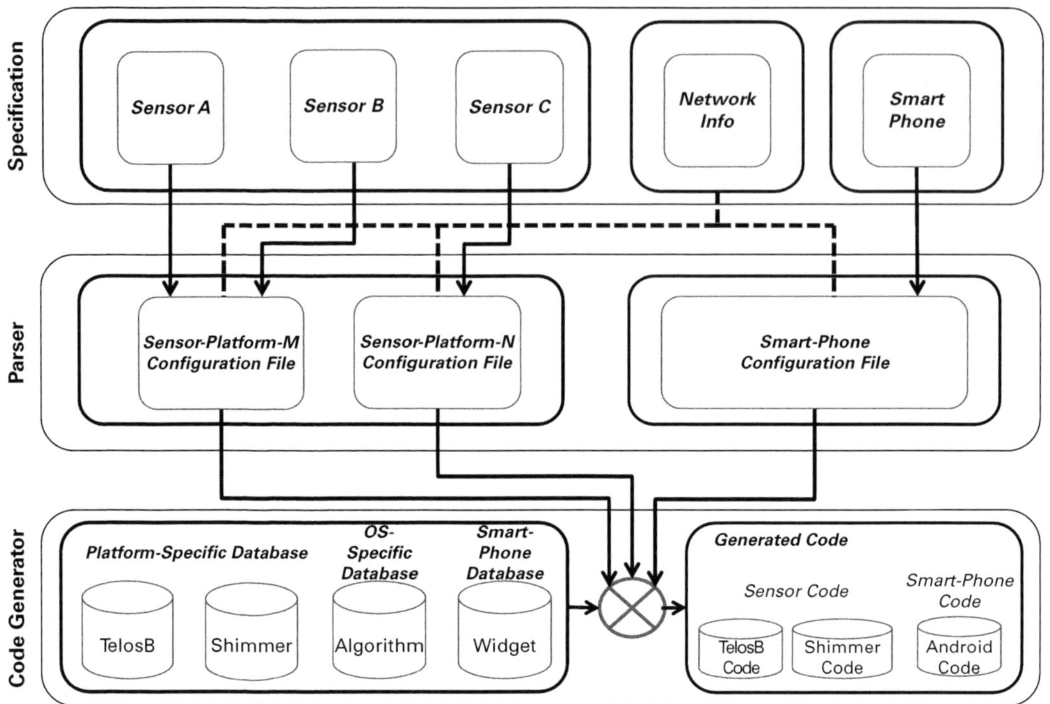

Figure 7.3   The architecture of Health-Dev.

Health-Dev is an automatic-code-generation tool that was developed at the IMPACT Lab at the ASU. Health-Dev considers code generation both for the smart phone and for the sensors. It is not limited to TinyOS-specific sensors but can also generate code for Linux-based sensors, such as iMote2, and other sensor-operating systems such as Arduino. Further, Health-Dev allows code generation for any Android-based smart phone. The architecture of Health-Dev is shown in Figure 7.3.

Health-Dev takes a high-level specification of the sensors and smart phones as input. This high-level specification is done using the AADL tool. The properties that can be specified using the AADL interface are shown in Table 7.1. The primary features of Health-Dev that set it apart from other code generators are (a) it is not TinyOS-specific, (b) it allows code generation for smart phones, (c) it supports programming of both Bluetooth and ZigBee protocol stacks, (d) it allows two-way communication between the smart phone and the sensors, and (e) it allows coding of physiological signal processing algorithms in sensors. The current state-of-the-art automatic code generators are, however, limited in several aspects. Generation of code for adaptive thresholding in sensors is still an area to be researched. Another area of interest is that of the over-the-air reprogramming of sensors. This requires rebuilding the kernel and making changes to the boot loader of the sensors. Current tools for automatic code generation do not support these functionalities.

Table 7.1 Specifiable properties in Health-Dev

Sensing	Computation	Communication	Phone
1. Node ID	1. Physiological processing (BSNBench, heart-rate calculator, ECG models)	1. Routing protocol (Bluetooth or ZigBee)	1. Buttons onclicks, text views
2. Platform		2. Destination and source address	2. Graphing variables
3. Sensor type		3. Packet contents	3. Execution sequences
4. Sampling frequency	2. Execution sequence	4. Radio duty cycle	4. Control commands to sensors

7.7 Data repositories

To validate any implementation of a BAN, experimental data are required. Since BANs deal with physiological data, repositories of different physiological signals are extremely useful for BAN researchers. In this regard, researchers throughout the world have made physiological data collected during the course of their projects available online. Table 7.2 lists databases of physiological signals, and gives a brief description of their contents.

7.8 Questions

Several BAN application examples and exercises are available online at http://impact.asu.edu/BANBook.html. Below we provide few simple exercises for you to get started with programming wireless sensors and smart phones. Although the following exercises recommend using TinyOS, TelosB, and Android systems, they can easily be done using any other equivalent wireless sensor network system.

1. Write a TinyOS program to display a 3-bit counter using TelosB LEDs.
2. Write a TinyOS program to
   (1) read the light sensor periodically
   (2) send the sensed sample (blink LED 2 whenever you send a packet)
   (3) if the light-sensor intensity goes below 10 units, stop the radio (turn LED 1 on)
   (4) when the light-sensor intensity goes back up over 10 units, restart the radio (turn LED 1 off)
   (5) go to step 2.
3. Write an Android app to continuously display collected physiological signals on a graph.
4. Write an Android app and the corresponding TinyOS code to enable Bluetooth communication between mobile devices and the sensor.

Table 7.2 Physiological signal repositories

Database name	Weblink	Contents
MIT BIH Physiobank	`http://www.physionet.org/`	ECG and PPG signals of thousands of patients suffering from different pathological conditions such as arrhythmia
Berlin Database of Emotional Speech (EmoDB)	`http://emotion-research.net/biblio/tuDatabase`	Ten actors (five female and five male) simulated emotions, producing ten utterances (five short and five longer sentences, in German), which could be used in everyday communication and are interpretable in terms of all applied emotions
IMPACT database	`http://impact.asu.edu/IMPACTDataset.zip`	PPG data of 16 volunteers with no apparent pathological conditions collected using Smithsoem fingertip pulse oximeters at 60 Hz
CASIA Gait Database	`http://www.cbsr.ia.ac.cn/english/Gait%20Databases.asp`	Four databases collected using different types of cameras including infra-red cameras with over 100 people on different terrains
UC Irvine EEG database	`http://kdd.ics.uci.edu/databases/eeg/eeg.html`	Data from a large study to examine EEG correlates of genetic predisposition to alcoholism, containing measurements from 64 electrodes placed on the scalp sampled at 256 Hz (3.9-ms epoch) for 1 s
Consolidated Human Activity Database	`http://www.epa.gov/chadnet1/`	Data obtained from pre-existing human activity studies that were collected at city, state, and national levels

5. Integrate a physiological sensor with a TelosB mote and develop an Android application for physiological sensing that collects the sensed data, processes them, and displays them on the Android platform.

8 Epilogue

A decade ago wireless sensor networks (WSNs), resulting primarily from developments in miniaturization and low-powered electronics, opened up the possibility of deploying computing capabilities ubiquitously. Not surprisingly, the last few years have seen the extension of this capability to the human body, leading to the development of body area networks (BANs), which are networks of medical devices and sensors worn on or implanted in the human body. They are used for monitoring and actuation purposes and typically applied in, but not limited to, medical settings. In this book we have aimed at providing a systematic description of how to design and develop safe, secure, and sustainable BANs. We have focused on ideas heretofore available only in scattered research articles and development guides for open-source sensor platforms. Our hope is to bring the latest technological developments in the domain of BANs to a wider audience.

Body area networks are becoming increasingly vital for nations and societies worldwide, especially in an attempt to reduce the burgeoning healthcare costs. In this book we have attempted to give a cohesive account of (i) their principal components, properties, and characteristics; (ii) the need for safe, secure, and sustainable design of BANs and the approaches available for addressing this need; and (iii) experiences with, and issues involved in, implementing actual BANs, drawing on lessons learnt from actual implementation. So far, the major focus of the BAN community has been on developing the hardware platforms and basic signal-processing techniques for BANs. Although this work is important, in writing this book we have been driven by our belief that it is now time to move beyond this platform-centric focus to issues that are important at a higher abstraction – namely in terms of ensuring the safety, security, and sustainability of BANs – and more broadly to enabling pervasive healthcare. A substantial gap exists in this regard. We believe that this book is a step towards bridging this gap.

The book has provided a unique perspective in designing safe, secure, and sustainable BANs. It has viewed these issues in the light of BANs being examples of cyber-physical systems (CPSes), which are environment-coupled systems that have the ability to monitor and control the environment they are a part of. To this end, we adopted a model-based approach for designing BANs taking into account their environment-coupled nature. Specifically, the book contains

- a model-based engineering approach to improve the safety of BANs, including a case-study featuring a safety-design and -analysis tool called BAND-AiDe to study the thermal effects of sensor operation on the human body;

- an environment-coupled approach to improve the security of BANs, including a case-study that utilizes physiological signals to enable key agreement between sensors, making trusted communication possible;
- an approach that utilizes models of various BAN architectures and energy sources, in conjunction, to design sustainable BANs, including a case-study that demonstrates the effectiveness of various energy-scavenging mechanisms in sustaining a health-monitoring BAN;
- an overview of available BAN programming paradigms, and how to go about conducting the design, analysis, and verification of BANs; and
- an overview of regulatory issues specific to BANs in various parts of the world.

The book has been written with advanced courses and graduate-level seminars in mind. We expect that it will allow students to gain a conceptual appreciation of BANs in general and, more specifically, using the model-based environment-coupled design methodology for designing them. The book will also be of interest to people interested in the up and coming field of CPSes who want an overview of the typical issues involved and how to go about designing them. Additionally, practitioners in the application area will find the book useful as a monograph on the new domain. Further, since this is a growing area of research, the appendix identifies a number of research groups involved with BANs. Readers are encouraged to visit their webpages in order to get an idea of the interesting research they are undertaking.

The future for BANs is bright. As the devices get miniaturized further, they will be deployed on the human body in large numbers, enabling newer and more advanced monitoring and actuation capabilities. However, given their form factor and the capability of individual sensors, it will be an increasingly difficult challenge to ensure that they are safe, secure, and sustainable. The model-based environment-coupled design methodology covered in this book, in our view, provides researchers and practitioners with tools and techniques for solving these problems, going forward to the next generation of BANs. That being said, much work still needs to be done to enhance the capabilities of model-based BAN design methodology, including dealing with the effects of complex physiological processes such as tissue growth (on implantable sensors) on their safe operation; removing the effects of topographic specificity from physiological-signal measurement, leading to potential physiological-signal-based secret generation; and characterizing the complex physical processes in the physical environment which affect scavenging and predicting the power available from a scavenging source for sustainability.

We sincerely hope that our predictions regarding the wider adoption of pervasive healthcare come to fruition, and that it becomes a driving force in bringing down the cost of healthcare and keeping the growing and aging world populace healthy.

May you live a long and healthy life, or, as they bless in Sanskrit – Ayushman Bhava!

Glossary

ASIC: Application-specific integrated circuit.

Architectural model: A representation of a system in terms of its components and the connections between them. The connections may indicate flow of data or control signals from one component to the other or simply a subcomponent relationship.

Architecture Analysis & Design Language (AADL): An architecture-description language standardized by the Society of Automotive Engineers. It is used to model the software and hardware components of embedded, real-time systems.

Assurance cases: Assurance cases represent a framework for arguing that evidence justifies a claim. They provide a means for convincing a third party, such as a regulator, that a particular claim is justified. They are currently used for evaluating medical devices and military avionics.

Asymmetric key cryptography: The form of cryptography whereby one key is used for encryption and another for decryption.

Authentication: Ensure that the system knows the identities of all the entities interacting with it, and vice versa.

Authorization: Ensure that any entity trying to access particular information from the system is able to access only that information to which they are entitled.

Availability: Ensure that any entity that should be able to use the data, services, and resources of the system is able to do so when required.

BAN-CPS: A BAN viewed from the perspective of cyber-physical systems.

BAN safety: Ensuring that physical side-effects of the operations of the sensors in the BAN remain within desired limits.

BAN security: Preventing unauthorized entities from viewing, accessing, or modifying data generated within the BAN.

BAN sustainability: Ensuring uninterrupted operation of the entire BAN.

BAND-AiDe: A tool that provides a uniform model-specification and -analysis platform enabling model-based engineering (i.e., both model development and analysis) of BANs.

Behavioral model: A representation of a system or a process as a black box, with inputs, outputs, and a transfer function specifying the relation between them.

Biometrics: A method for uniquely identifying humans in terms of intrinsic physical or behavioral traits. Examples include fingerprints and iris images.

Biosensors: Physical, chemical, and biological sensors combined with integrated circuits with applications in the biomedical domain such as health monitoring, prosthesis, and rehabilitation.

Bluetooth: A wireless communication protocol intended for one-hop master–slave communication.

Body sensor network/body area network (BSN/BAN): A collection of ambient sensors and biosensors organized as a network for coordinated data collection and actuation. BANs are also referred to as BAN-CPSes.

BSNBench: A benchmarking suite intended specifically to evaluate BANs with respect to different design coordinates.

CPS-Sec: A class of security solutions that use input from the surrounding physical processes to operate.

Cyber-physical systems (CPSes): A class of distributed systems that have a very tight coupling between the system's computational and physical elements.

Data confidentiality: Ensuring that all sensitive information generated within the system is disclosed only to those who are supposed to see it.

Data integrity: Ensuring that all information generated and exchanged during the system's operation is accurate and complete, without any alterations.

Denial of service: A form of attack that compromises the availability of a system. Examples include radio-channel jamming.

Design coordinate: A property of the BAN, a change of which can be attributed to a specific component in the sensor platform.

Design space: The coordinate space formed by representing design coordinates as coordinate axes.

Duty cycle: The time during which a system is active expressed as a percentage of the total time for which it is under consideration.

Eavesdropping: A form of passive attack whereby a malicious entity overhears communication between two legitimate entities within a system.

Electrocardiogram (ECG): A measure of the electrical activity of the heart over a period of time.

Electronic patient record (EPR): An individual's health information in electronic format. The EPR has been designed to replace today's paper-based records, which are cumbersome to manage. They are used to facilitate storage of, and access to, patient data (through the Internet), improve the availability of all aspects of patient data at a single location, and provide intelligent indexing and data-mining capabilities relating to health data.

Energy-neutral: Energy-neutrality of a system essentially means that the system consumes as much energy as it harvests.

Energy scavenging: The process of extracting energy from ambient sources such as solar, thermal, wind, movement, and so on.

Event: A periodically or randomly occurring phenomenon detected by a sensor in a BAN.

Failure modes and effects analysis (FMEA): An operations-management term for analyzing the potential failure modes within a system and classifying them by severity and likelihood of occurrence.

False negative: A test that fails to reject a false null hypothesis.

False positive: A test that rejects a true null hypothesis.

Fast Fourier transform (FFT): An efficient algorithm to compute the discrete Fourier transform (DFT), which transforms a signal from the time domain to the frequency domain.

Formal model: A representation of a system's operation in terms of discrete states and transitions between them. Formal models are of different types – finite-state automata, timed automata, and hybrid systems.

FPGA: Field-programmable gate array.

Fuzzy vault: The way of hiding a secret using a set of values, say A, in such a manner that it can be un-hidden with another set of values B, provided that A and B share a certain number of common values, i.e., $A \cap B > \Delta$.

Generative model: A model of a physiological signal that, when provided with the correct inputs, can regenerate the signal for a given physiological condition of a given patient.

Hardware adaptation layer (HAL): An application-specific abstraction of the hardware components of a sensor platform.

Hardware interface layer (HIL): An application-independent abstraction of the hardware components of a sensor platform.

Hardware presentation layer (HPL): An abstraction of the hardware components of a sensor that provides very basic functionalities for starting and stopping the component.

Hazard analysis: A structured tool for demonstrating that all hazards faced by a system in a specific context are accounted for and that their effects have been mitigated.

Healthcare delivery model: The steps a person has to go through in the process of obtaining care. The traditional model involves four steps: detect symptoms, and then visit a medical caregiver, who performs diagnosis and facilitates treatment.

Health Information Portability and Accountability Act (HIPAA): Some 1996 legislation that protects health-insurance coverage for workers and their families when they change or lose their jobs. Further, a portion of the legislation known as the Administrative Simplification (AS) requires the establishment of national standards for electronic healthcare transactions and national identifiers for providers, health-insurance plans, and employers. The provisions of the Administration Simplification also address the security and privacy of health data.

Intended interaction: The usage of information from the physical environment for performing useful computing operations.

Key agreement: The process by which cryptographic keys are distributed between entities that want to communicate in a confidential and integrity-protected manner.

Mean time before failure (MTBF): The frequency with which engineered components fail. Also known as the failure rate.

Model: A model is an abstract representation of a system or a process.

Model-based engineering: A way of developing systems that satisfy design requirements. The idea is to develop models that capture the functional aspects of the systems, and then analyze them formally to prove that they satisfy the requirements.

Nonce: A number used in cryptographic protocols in order to maintain transaction freshness. A nonce must be different for every protocol run.

Pervasive healthcare: The use of pervasive computing technologies for day-to-day healthcare management to enable real-time, continuous patient monitoring.

Photoplethysmogram (PPG): A measure of the distension of the arteries as a result of the activity of the heart over a period of time. It is measured using pulse oximeters.

Pre-market approval (PMA): An FDA review process for evaluating the safety and effectiveness of class III medical devices.

Privacy: Protection from unauthorized disclosure of data.

Region of impact (ROIm): Assuming that any interaction of the computing unit with the physical world will take place within a bounded region, the ROIm construct models the un-intentional interactions.

Region of interest (ROIn): Assuming that any interaction of the computing unit with the physical world will take place within a bounded region, the ROIn construct models the intentional interactions.

Role-based access control (RBAC): An access-control mechanism that groups users in terms of the tasks they perform within the system, called roles, and provides access to the roles, instead of to individuals.

Spatial–temporal hybrid automata (STHA): A formal model in which, a state represents the system's properties and their variations at a particular time in a particular space. The state variables in such a formal model vary in a continuous domain both in time and in space, and their variation should be governed by spatio-temporal partial differential equations.

Spoofing: A form of attack whereby a malicious entity pretends to be an entity that it is not when it is interacting with the system. An extreme form of this attack is the *Sybil* attack, in which the malicious entity presents itself with multiple identities to a system.

Symmetric-key cryptography: The form of cryptography in which the same key is used both for encryption and for decryption.

Task: Threads in TinyOS that are used for long-running computations in the sensor.

Telemedicine: The remote diagnosis and treatment of patients using communication technologies.

Topographic specificity: The spatial variation in physiological parameters which is observed over the body. This causes dissimilar values of correlation coefficients to be measured for the same physiological signals when they are synchronously measured at two different locations on the body.

Threat model: A systematic taxonomy of potential threats that a system faces in various contexts.

Time-division multiple access: A channel-access scheme for networks with shared medium. The scheme divides the available time into slots and allocates each of them to entities that want to communicate. This avoids contention for channels; however, it requires strict time synchronization.

TinyOS: A single-application sensor-node operating system.

Trust: The subjective expectation that an entity will behave in a particular manner.

Unintended interaction: The side-effects of operation of the computing units on the physical environment.

Validation: The process of establishing that a model replicates the behavior of a real system with the desired accuracy.

Verification: The process of determining whether the model of a system meets the requirements set forth by the designer.

Window of opportunity: The duration after the occurrence of a criticality within which all the effects of the criticality can be mitigated successfully. It varies according to the criticalities present.

ZigBee: A wireless communication protocol intended for self-healing mesh networking.

Appendix: Publication venues, academic research groups, and funding agencies

Body area networks (BANs) are increasingly becoming a topic of great interest for researchers. Researchers are involved in the development of cutting-edge hardware for BANs, and of their software infrastructure, using BANs in medical, sports, and entertainment applications, and building theoretical background for BAN design and verification. For the dissemination of this precious knowledge several prestigious journals and conferences have come into being. Pre-eminent among them are ACM Wireless Health (`http://www.wirelesshealth2012.org/`) and IEEE BSN (`http://www.bsn2012.org/`). There are many other conferences and journals that publish research articles on BSNs. Here is a list of a few of them: IEEE Milcom (`http://www.milcom.org/`), IEEE Infocom (`http://www.ieee-infocom.org/`), Percom (`http://www.percom.org/`), IEEE EMBC (`http://embc2012.embs.org/`), and ACM MSWiM (`http://mswimconf.com/2012/`) are important conferences; while *ACM TECS* (`http://acmtecs.acm.org/`), *ACM TOSN* (`https://sites.google.com/site/acmtosn/`), *IEEE TON* (`http://www.ton.seas.upenn.edu/`), *IEEE Proceedings* (`http://ieeexplore.ieee.org/xpl/RecentIssue.jsp?punumber=5`), and *IEEE TITB* (`http://bme.ee.cuhk.edu.hk/TITB/`) are notable journals.

There are many academic research groups that are working on various hardware and software aspects of BANs. Specifically, the following academic research groups are involved in research related to BAN software: the IMPACT Lab at Arizona State University (`http://bme.ee.cuhk.edu.hk/TITB/`), the Media Labs at MIT (`http://www.media.mit.edu/`), the Center for Wireless Health at the University of Virginia (`http://wirelesshealth.virginia.edu/`), the ESSP Lab at the University of Texas, Dallas (`http://wirelesshealth.virginia.edu/`), the Wireless Life Sciences Alliances at the University of California, Los Angeles (`http://www.wirelesslifesciences.org/`), Imperial College London (`http://www3.imperial.ac.uk/`), the NSL at the University of Washington, the Harvard Sensor Networks Lab, and the UAV Center for Wireless Health (`http://wirelesshealth.virginia.edu/`).

The federal funding agencies in the USA such as the National Institutes for Health (NIH) (`http://www.nih.gov/`) and the National Science Foundation (NSF) (`http://www.nsf.gov/`) have several programs to support research into BANs. There are also several industrial concerns such as Intel Corp. and Google Inc. that fund research in this area.

References

[1] Aging Report 2006. The impact of the aging population on the health workforce in the United States: summary of key findings. Center for Health Workforce Studies School of Public Health, University at Albany, 2006.

[2] *World Population Ageing: 1950–2050*. United Nations, Department of Economic and Social Affairs, Population Division.

[3] V. Stanford. Pervasive health care applications face tough security challenges. *IEEE Pervasive Computing*, 1(2):8–12, 2002.

[4] Updated national health expenditure projections 2009–2019. `http://www.cms.gov/NationalHealthExpendData/downloads/NHEProjections2009to2019.pdf`, Sep. 2010.

[5] iTunes. Calorie tracker. `http://itunes.apple.com/us/app/calorie-tracker-livestrong.com/id295305241?mt=8`.

[6] iTunes. Lose the belly. `http://itunes.apple.com/us/app/lose-belly-weight-loss-for/id333182979?mt=8`.

[7] AppBrain. Instant heart rate. `http://www.appbrain.com/app/instant-heart-rate/si.modula.android.instantheartrate`.

[8] iTunes. Nursing health assessment. `http://itunes.apple.com/us/app/nursing-health-assessment/id403625924?mt=8`.

[9] Singularity Health Law. FDA to regulate minor subset of smart phone medical device apps. `http://gregpiche.typepad.com/blog/2011/09/fda-to-regulate-minor-subset-of-smartphone-medical-device-applications.html`.

[10] U. Varshney. Pervasive healthcare. *IEEE Computer*, 36(12):138–140, 2003.

[11] K. Venkatasubramanian, S. Nabar, S. K. S. Gupta, and R. Poovendran. Cyber physical security solutions for pervasive health monitoring systems, in *E-Healthcare Systems and Wireless Communications: Current and Future Challenges*, ed. M. Watfa. IGI Global, pages 143–162, 2012.

[12] M. Sung, C. Marci, and A. Pentland. Wearable feedback systems for rehabilitation. *Journal of Neuroengineering and Rehabilitation*, 2:17, June 2005.

[13] U. Anliker, J. A. Ward, P. Lukowicz *et al.* Amon: A wearable multiparameter medical monitoring and alert system. *IEEE Transactions on Information Technology and Biomedicine*, 8:415–427, Dec. 2004.

[14] C. Mundt, K. N. Montgomery, U. E. Udoh *et al.* A multi-parameter wearable physiological monitoring system for space and terrestrial applications. *IEEE Transactions on Information Technology and Biomedicine*, 9:382–391, Sep. 2005.

[15] R. Paradiso, G. Loriga, and N. Taccini. A wearable health care system based on knitted integral sensors. *IEEE Transactions on Information Technology and Biomedicine*, 9:337–344, Sep. 2005.

[16] J. Habetha. The MyHeart project – fighting cardiovascular diseases by prevention and early diagnosis, in *Proceedings of the 28th Annual International Conference of the IEEE Engineering in Medicine and Biology Society*, pages 6746–6749, 2006. IEEE.

[17] E. P. Scilingo, A. Gemignami, R. Paradiso *et al.* Performance evaluation of sensing fabrics for monitoring physiological and biomechanical variables. *IEEE Transactions on Information Technology and Biomedicine*, 9:345–352, Sep. 2005.

[18] A. Lymperis and R. Paradiso. Smart and interactive textile enabling wearable personal applications: R&D state of the art and future challenges, in *Proceedings of the 30th Annual International Conference of the IEEE Engineering in Medicine and Biology Society*, pages 5270–5273, 2008. IEEE.

[19] M. D. Rienzo, F. Rizzo, G. Parati *et al.* Magic system: a new textile-based wearable device for biological signal monitoring applicability in daily life and clinical setting, in *Proceedings of the 27th Annual International Conference of the IEEE Engineering in Medicine and Biology Society*, pages 7167–7169, 2005. IEEE.

[20] P. S. Pandian, K. Mohanavelu, K. P. Safeer *et al.* Smart vest: wearable multiparameter remote physiological monitoring system. *Medical Engineering and Physics*, 30:466–477, May 2008.

[21] S. Park and S. Jayaraman. Smart textile-based wearable biomedical systems: a transition plan for research to reality. *IEEE Transactions on Information Technology and Biomedicine*, 14(1):86–92, Jan. 2010.

[22] V. Shnayder, B. R. Chen, K. Lorincz, T. R. F. Fulford-Jones, and M. Welsh. Sensor networks for medical care. Technical report TR-08-05, Division of Engineering and Applied Science, Harvard University, Cambridge, MA, 2005.

[23] A. Wood, G. Virone, T. Doan *et al.* Alarm-net: wireless sensor networks for assisted-living and residential monitoring. Technical report CS-2006-11, Department of Computer Science, University of Virginia, 2006.

[24] B. Gyselinckx, J. Penders, and R. Vullers. Potential and challenges of body area networks for cardiac monitoring. *Journal of Electrocardiology*, 40:S165–S168, Nov. 2007.

[25] N. Loew, K.-J. Winzer, G. Becher *et al.* Medical sensors of the BASUMA body sensor network, in *Proceedings of the 4th International Workshop on Wearable Implantable BSN*, pages 171–176, May 2007.

[26] Z. Jin, J. Oresko, S Huang, and A. C. Cheng. Hearttogo: a personalized medicine technology for cardiovascular disease prevention and detection, in *Proceedings of the IEEE/NIH LiSSA*, pages 80–83, 2009. IEEE/NIH.

[27] I. F. Akyildiz, W. Su, Y. Sankarasubramaniam, and E. Cayirci. Wireless sensor networks: a survey. *Computer Networks*, 38:393–422, 2002.

[28] E. Jovanov, D. Raskovic, J. Price *et al.* Patient monitoring using personal area networks of wireless intelligent sensors. *Biomedical Sciences Instrumentation*, 37:373–378, 2001.

[29] L. Schwiebert, S. K. Gupta, and J. Weinmann. Research challenges in wireless networks of biomedical sensors, in *MobiCom '01: Proceedings of the 7th Annual International Conference on Mobile Computing and Networking*, pages 151–165, New York, NY, 2001. ACM.

[30] L. Schwiebert, S. K. S. Gupta, P. Siy, G. Auner, and G. Abrams. A biomedical smart sensor for the visually impaired, in *IEEE Sensors 2002*, pages 11–14, 2002. IEEE.

[31] Medical Electronics Design magazine. Medical device networks. `http:// www.medicalelectronicsdesign.com/article/medical-device- network-control-standards`.

[32] J. A. Paradiso and T. Starner. Energy scavenging for mobile and wireless electronics. *IEEE Pervasive Computing*, 4(1):18–27, Jan.–Mar. 2005.

[33] D. Bhatia, S. Bairagi, S. Goel, and M. Jangra. Pacemakers charging using body energy. *Journal of Pharmacology and Bioallied Sciences*, 2: 51–54, 2010.

[34] N. Kern and B. Schiele. Multi-sensor activity context detection for wearable computing, in *Proceedings of the European Symposium on Ambient Intelligence*, 2003.

[35] K. V. Laerhoven and H. W. Gellersen. Spine versus Porcupine: a study in distributed wearable activity recognition, in *Proceedings of the 8th International Symposium on Wearable Computers*, pages 142–149, 2004.

[36] J. Elson, L. Girod, and D. Estrin. Fine-grained network time synchronization using reference broadcasts, in *Proceedings of the 5th Symposium on Operating Systems Design and Implementation*, pages 147–163, 2002.

[37] S. Ganeriwal, S. Capkun, C. Han, and M. Srivastava. Secure time synchronization service for sensor networks, in *Proceedings of the 4th ACM Workshop on Wireless Security*, 2005. ACM.

[38] A. Alomainy, Y. Hao, A. Owadally *et al.* Statistical analysis and performance evaluation for on-body radio propagation with microstrip patch antennas. *IEEE Transactions on Antennas and Propagation*, 55(1):245–248, 2007.

[39] S. Cotton and W. Scanlon. An experimental investigation into influence of user state and environment on fading characteristics in wireless body area networks at 2.45 GHz. *IEEE Transactions on Wireless Communications*, 8(1):6–12, 2009.

[40] B. Zhen, M. Kim, J.-I. Takada, and R. Kohno. Characterization and modeling of dynamic on-body propagation at 4.5 GHz. *IEEE Journal of Antennas and Wireless Propagation Letters*, 8:1263–1267, 2009.

[41] T. G. Zimmerman. Personal area networks: near-field intrabody communication. *IBM Systems Journal*, 35(3–4):609–617, 1996.

[42] M. E. Morris. Social networks as health feedback displays. *IEEE Internet Computing*, 9(5):29–37, 2005.

[43] P. McSharry, G. Clifford, L. Tarassenko, and L. Smith. A dynamical model for generating synthetic electrocardiogram signals. *IEEE Transactions on Biomedical Engineering*, 50(3):289–294, 2003.

[44] J. Allen. Photoplethysmography and its application in clinical physiological measurement. *Physiological Measurement*, 28:R1, 2007.

[45] A. Reisner, P. A. Shaltis, D. McCombie, and H. H. Asada. Utility of the photoplethysmogram in circulatory monitoring. *Anesthesiology*, 108(5):950–958, 2008.

[46] S. C. Millasseau, J. M. Ritter, K. Takazawa, and P. J. Chowienczyk, Contour analysis of the photoplethysmographic pulse measured at the finger. *Journal of Hypertension*, 24(8):1449–1456, 2006.

[47] N. Selvaraj, A. K. Jaryal, J. Santhosh, K. K. Deepak, and S. Anand. Assessment of heart rate variability derived from finger-tip photoplethysmography as compared to electrocardiography. *Journal of Medical Engineering & Technology*, 32(6):479–484, 2008.

[48] V. Crabtree and P. Smith. Physiological models of the human vasculature and photoplethysmography. Technical report, Electronic Systems and Control Division Research, Department of Electronic and Electrical Engineering, Loughborough University, pages 60–63, 2003.

[49] University of Pennsylvania. Generic infusion pump project. http://rtg.cis.upenn.edu/gip.php3.

[50] D. Wada and D. Ward. The hybrid model: a new pharmacokinetic model for computer-controlled infusion pumps. *IEEE Transactions on Biomedical Engineering*, 41(2):134–142, Feb. 1994.

[51] Y. Ozier, P. Guéret, F. Jardin *et al.* Two-dimensional echocardiographic demonstration of acute myocardial depression in septic shock. *Critical Care Medicine*, 12(7):596–599, 1984.

[52] F. Adelstein, S. K. S. Gupta, G. Richard, and L. Schwiebert. *Fundamentals of Mobile and Pervasive Computing*. McGraw Hill, 2004.

[53] K. Venkatasubramanian, G. Deng, T. Mukherjee *et al.* Ayushman: a wireless sensor network based health monitoring infrastructure and testbed, in *Distributed Computing in Sensor Systems*, pages 406–407, Springer, 2005.

[54] ISO 60601 safety standard. `http://www.iso.org/iso/iso_catalogue/catalogue_tc/catalogue_detail.htm\?csnumber=45605`.

[55] R. Jetley, S. P. Iyer, and P. L. Jones. A formal methods approach to medical device review. *Computer*, 39(4):61–67, 2006.

[56] D. E. Arney, R. Jetley, P. Jones *et al.* Generic infusion pump hazard analysis and safety requirements version 1.0, Technical report, Department of Computer & Information Science, University of Pennsylvania, 2009.

[57] D. Halperin, T. S. Heydt-Benjamin, B. Ransford *et al.* Pacemakers and implantable cardiac defibrillators: software radio attacks and zero-power defenses, in *Proceedings of the IEEE Symposium on Security and Privacy*, 2008. IEEE.

[58] A. Kansal, J. Hsu, M. Srivastava, and V. Raghunathan. Harvesting aware power management for sensor networks, in *Proceedings of the 43rd annual Design Automation Conference, DAC '06*, pages 651–656, 2006.

[59] H. H. Pennes. Analysis of tissue and arterial blood temperature in the resting human forearm. *Journal of Applied Physiology*, 1(1):93–122, 1948.

[60] R. N. Maini, F. C. Breedveld, J. R. Kalden *et al.* Therapeutic efficacy of multiple intravenous infusions of anti-tumor necrosis factor, a monoclonal antibody, combined with low-dose weekly methotrexate in rheumatoid arthritis. *Arthritis and Rheumatism*, 41(9):1552–1563, 1998.

[61] Q. Tang, G. Varsamopoulos, and S. K. S. Gupta. Energy-efficient thermal-aware task scheduling for homogeneous high-performance computing data centers: a cyber-physical approach. *IEEE Transactions on Parallel and Distributed Systems, Special Issue on Power-Aware Parallel and Distributed Systems (TPDS/PAPADS)*, 11(19):1458–1472, Nov. 2008.

[62] Safe Medical Devices Act. `http://www.fda.gov/cdrh/devadvice/312.html`.

[63] D. Arney, K. K. Venkatasubramanian, O. Sokolsky, and I. Lee. Biomedical devices and systems security, in *Proceedings of the 33rd Annual International Conference of the IEEE Engineering in Medicine and Biology Society*, 2011. IEEE.

[64] K. Venkatasubramanian, T. Mukherjee, and S. K. S. Gupta. CAAC – an adaptive and proactive access control approach for emergencies for smart infrastructures. *ACM Transactions on Autonomous and Adaptive Systems, Special Issue on Adaptive Security*, 2012.

[65] T. Mukherjee, K. Venkatasubramanian, and S. Gupta. Performance modeling of critical event management for ubiquitous computing applications, in *MSWiM '06: Proceedings of the 9th ACM International Symposium on Modeling, Analysis and Simulation of Wireless and Mobile Systems*, pages 12–19, 2006. ACM.

[66] V. Gehlot and E. B. Sloane. Ensuring patient safety in wireless medical device networks. *Computer*, 39:54–60, Apr. 2006.

[67] A. Banerjee and S. K. S. Gupta. Your mobility can be injurious to your health: analyzing pervasive health monitoring systems under dynamic context changes, in *Proceedings of the 10th IEEE Conference on Pervasive Computing (PerCom)*, pages 39–47, 2012. IEEE.

[68] W. R. Heinzelman, A. Chandrakasan, and H. Balakrishnan. Energy-efficient communication protocol for wireless microsensor networks, in *HICSS '00: Proceedings of the 33rd Hawaii International Conference on System Sciences*, page 8020, Washington, DC, 2000. IEEE Computer Society.

[69] Q. Tang, N. Tummala, S. K. S. Gupta, and L. Schwiebert. Communication scheduling to minimize thermal effects of implanted biosensor networks in homogeneous tissue. *IEEE Transactions on Biomedical Engineering*, 52(7):1285–1294, July 2005.

[70] L. Bleris and M. Kothare. Implementation of model predictive control for glucose regulation on a general purpose microprocessor, in *Decision and Control, 2005 and 2005 44th IEEE Conference on European Control Conference, CDC-ECC '05*, pages 5162–5167, 2005. IEEE.

[71] A. Banerjee, K. Venkatasubramanian, T. Mukherjee, and S. Gupta. Ensuring safety, security, and sustainability of mission-critical cyber-physical systems. *Proceedings of the IEEE*, 100(1):283–299, Jan. 2012.

[72] D. G. M. Greenhalgh, M. B. R. Lawless, B. B. Chew *et al.* Temperature threshold for burn injury: an oximeter safety study. *Journal of Burn Care and Rehabilitation*, 25(5):411–415, 2004.

[73] S. Weininger, J. Pfefer, and I. Chang. Factors to consider in a risk analysis for safe surface temperature, in *2005 IEEE Symposium on Product Safety Engineering*, pages 83–91, 2005. IEEE.

[74] Z. Jiang, M. Pajic, A. Connolly, S. Dixit, and R. Mangharam. Real-time heart model for implantable cardiac device validation and verification, in *ECRTS*, pages 239–248, 2010.

[75] D. Arney, M. Pajic, J. M. Goldman *et al.* Toward patient safety in closed-loop medical device systems, in *ICCPS '10: Proceedings of the 1st ACM/IEEE International Conference on Cyber-Physical Systems*, pages 139–148, New York, NY, 2010. ACM.

[76] P. W. Tuinenga. *Spice: A Guide to Circuit Simulation and Analysis Using PSpice.* Prentice Hall, 1991.

[77] G.-M. Elena and M. José. Argospe: model-based software performance engineering, in *ICATPN*, pages 401–410, 2006.

[78] V. Prasad, T. Yan, P. Jayachandran, *et al.* ANDES: an analysis-based design tool for wireless sensor networks, in *28th IEEE International Real-Time Systems Symposium, RTSS 2007*, pages 203–213, 2007. IEEE.

[79] S. Coleri M. Ergen, and T. J. Koo. Lifetime analysis of a sensor network with hybrid automata modelling, in *WSNA '02: Proceedings of the 1st ACM International Workshop on Wireless Sensor Networks and Applications*, pages 98–104, New York, NY, 2002. ACM.

[80] A. Banerjee, S. Kandula, T. Mukherjee, and S. K. S. Gupta. BAND-AiDe: a tool for cyber-physical oriented analysis and design of body area networks and devices. *ACM Transactions on Embedded Computer Systems*, 11(S2):49-1–49-29, Aug. 2012.

[81] A. Bhave, B. Krogh, D. Garlan, and B. Schmerl. View consistency in architectures for cyber-physical systems, in *Proceedings of the 2nd ACM/IEEE International Conference on Cyber-Physical Systems*, Apr. 2011. ACM.

[82] A. Banerjee, K. Venkatasubramanian, and S. K. S. Gupta. Challenges of implementing cyber-physical security solutions in body area networks, in *Proceedings of the International Conference on Body Area Networks*, 18 pages, 2009.

[83] F. C. J. Henriques and A. R. Moritz. Studies of thermal injury: I. The conduction of heat to and through skin and the temperatures attained therein. A theoretical and an experimental investigation. *American Journal of Pathology*, 530–549, July 1947.

[84] K. K. Venkatasubramanian, A. Banerjee, and S. K. S. Gupta. Green and sustainable cyber-physical security solutions for body area networks, in *BSN '09: Proceedings of the 2009 Sixth International Workshop on Wearable and Implantable Body Sensor Networks*, pages 240–245, Washington, DC, 2009. IEEE Computer Society.

[85] D. Halperin, T. S. Heydt-Benjamin, K. Fu, T. Kohno, and W. H. Maisel. Security and privacy for implantable medical devices. *IEEE Pervasive Computing*, 7(1):30–39, 2008.

[86] G. Frehse. Phaver: algorithmic verification of hybrid systems past Hytech, in *HSCC*, pages 258–273, 2005.

[87] D. Paul, L. Nathan, Y. Bazhang, M. Yvonne, and F. Moussy. Study of the effects of tissue reactions on the function of implanted glucose sensors. *Journal of Biomedical Materials Research Part A*, 85(3):699–706, 2007.

[88] M. Malisoff and F. Mazenc. On control-Lyapunov functions for hybrid time-varying systems, in *Proceedings of the 45th IEEE Conference on Decision & Control*, pages 3265–3270, San Diego, CA, 2006. IEEE.

[89] M. Bishop. *Computer Security: Art and Science*. Addison-Wesley Professional, 1st edition, 2002.

[90] C. Kaufman, R. Perlman, and M. Speciner. *Network Security: Private Communication in a Public World*. Prentice Hall, 2nd edition, 2002.

[91] HIPAA Report 2003. Summary of HIPAA Health Insurance Probability and Accountability Act. US Department of Health and Human Service, May 2003.

[92] K. Venkatasubramanian, A. Banerjee, and S. K. S. Gupta. EKG-based key agreement in body sensor networks, in *Proceedings of the 2nd Workshop on Mission Critical Networks*, pages 1–6, 2008.

[93] L. Eschenauer and V. D. Gligor. A key-management scheme for distributed sensor networks, in *Proceedings of the 9th ACM Conference on Computer and Communications Security*, pages 41–47, Nov. 2002.

[94] S. Zhu, S. Setia, and S. Jajodia. LEAP+: efficient security mechanisms for large-scale distributed sensor networks. *ACM Transactions on Sensor Networks*, 2(4):500–528, Nov. 2006.

[95] D. J. Malan, M. Welsh, and M. D. Smith. A public-key infrastructure for key distribution in TinyOS based on elliptic curve cryptography, in *Proceedings of the IEEE 2nd International Conference on Sensors and Ad Hoc Communications and Networks*, pages 71–80, 2004. IEEE.

[96] Q. Wang, K. Ren, W. Lou, and Y. Zhang. Dependable and secure sensor data storage with dynamic integrity assurance, in *Proceedings of INFOCOM 2009*, pages 954–962, 2009. IEEE.

[97] A. K. Ghosh and T. M. Swaminatha. Software security and privacy risks in mobile e-commerce. *Communications of the ACM*, 44:51–57, Feb. 2001.

[98] G. Portokalidis, P. Homburg, K. Anagnostakis, and H. Bos. Paranoid android: versatile protection for smartphones, in *Proceedings of the 26th Annual Computer Security Applications Conference, ACSAC '10*, pages 347–356, New York, NY, 2010. ACM.

[99] C. Wang, Q. Wang, K. Ren, and W. Lou. Ensuring data storage security in cloud computing, in *17th International Workshop on Quality of Service, 2009. IWQoS*, pages 1–9, 2009.

[100] Q. Wang, C. Wang, J. Li, K. Ren, and W. Lou. Enabling public verifiability and data dynamics for storage security in cloud computing, in *Computer Security, ESORICS 2009*, pages 355–370, 2009. Springer.

[101] C. Wang, Q. Wang, K. Ren, and W. Lou. Privacy-preserving public auditing for data storage security in cloud computing, in *Proceedings of INFOCOM 2010*, pages 1–9, 2010. IEEE.

[102] S. K. S. Gupta, T. Mukherjee, and K. Venkatasubramanian. Criticality aware access control model for pervasive applications, in *Proceedings of the 4th IEEE Conference on Pervasive Computing (PerCom)*, 2006. IEEE.

[103] D. F. Ferraiolo, J. F. Barkley, and R. Chandramouli. *Comparing Authorization Management Cost for Identity-Based and Role-Based Access Control*, 1999. National Institute of Standards and Technology White Paper.

[104] A. Ferreira, R. Cruz-Correia, L. Antunes *et al.* How to break access control in a controlled manner, in *Proceedings of the Ninteenth Symposium on Computer-Based Medical Systems*, pages 847–854, June 2006. IEEE.

[105] A. Corradi, R. Montanari, and D. Tibaldi. Context-based access control management in ubiquitous environments, in *Proceedings of the Third International Symposium on Network Computing and Applications*, pages 253–260, Sep. 2004. IEEE.

[106] M. J. Covington, W. Long, and S. Srinivasan. Secure context-aware applications using environmental roles, in *Proceedings of the Sixth ACM Symposium on Access Control Models and Technology*, pages 10–20, May 2001. ACM.

[107] H. Chan, A. Perrig, and D. Song. Random key predistribution schemes for sensor network, in *Proceedings of the IEEE Symposium of Research in Security and Privacy*, pages 197–213, May 2003. IEEE.

[108] W. Du, J. Deng, Y. S. Han *et al.* A pairwise key predistribution scheme for wireless sensor networks. *ACM Transactions on Information Systems Security*, 8(2):228–258, 2005.

[109] D. Liu and P. Ning. Establishing pairwise keys in distributed sensor networks, in *Proceedings of the 10th ACM Conference on Computer and Communications Security*, pages 52–61, 2003. ACM.

[110] R. D. Pietro, L. V. Mancini, and A. Mei. Random key assignment for secure wireless sensor networks, in *Proceedings of the ACM Workshop on Security of Ad Hoc and Sensor Networks*, pages 62–71, 2003. ACM.

[111] B. Lai, S. Kim, and I. Verbauwhede. Scalable session key construction protocol for wireless sensor networks, in *Proceedings of IEEE Workshop on Large Scale Real-Time and Embedded Systems*, 2002. IEEE.

[112] A. Perrig, R. Szewczyk, V. Wen, D. Culler, and D. Tygar. SPINS: Security Protocol for Sensor Networks. *Wireless Networks*, 8(5):521–534, Sep. 2002.

[113] Q. Huang, J. Cukier, H. Kobayashi, B. Liu, and J. Zhang. Fast authenticated key establishment protocols for self-organizing sensor networks, in *Proceedings of the 2nd ACM International Conference on Wireless Sensor Networks and Applications*, pages 141–150, 2003. ACM.

[114] C. Kuo, M. Luk, R. Negi, and A. Perrig. Message-in-a-bottle: user-friendly and secure key deployment for sensor nodes, in *Proceedings of the ACM Conference on Embedded Networked Sensor System (SenSys 2007)*, 2007. ACM.

[115] F. Stajano and R. Anderson. The resurrecting duckling: security issues for ad-hoc wireless networks, in *Proceedings of the 7th International Workshop on Security Protocols*, pages 172–194, 1999.

[116] Y. Sutcu, H. T. Sencar, and N. Memon. A secure biometric authentication scheme based on robust hashing, in *Proceedings of the 7th Workshop on Multimedia and Security, MM & Sec '05*, pages 111–116, New York, NY, 2005. ACM.

[117] C. McWilliams. The biophysical properties of the transdermal measurement. `http://www.electrodermology.com/biophysprop.htm`, 2003. International Society of Electrodermologists.

[118] A. Juels and M. Sudan. A fuzzy vault scheme, in *Proceedings of the IEEE International Symposium on Information Theory*, page 408, 2002.

[119] S. Cherukuri, K. Venkatasubramanian, and S. K. S. Gupta. BioSec: a biometric based approach for securing communication in wireless networks of biosensors implanted in the human body, in *Proceedings of the Wireless Security and Privacy Workshop 2003*, pages 432–439, Oct. 2003.

[120] U. Uludag, S. Pankanti, and A. K. Jain. Fuzzy vault for fingerprints, in *Proceedings of Audio- and Video-based Biometric Person Authentication*, pages 310–319, 2005.

[121] A. D. Droitcour. Non-contact measurement of heart and respiration rates with a single-chip microwave Doppler radar, 2006. PhD Thesis, Stanford University.

[122] E. F. Greneker. Radar sensing of heartbeat and respiration at a distance with applications of the technology. *IEE Radar*, 449:150–154, 1997.

[123] H. Ibrahim, A. Ilinca, and J. Perron. Energy storage systems – characteristics and comparisons. *Renewable and Sustainable Energy Reviews*, 12(5):1221–1250, 2008.

[124] H. Lund and G. Salgi. The role of compressed air energy storage (CAES) in future sustainable energy systems. *Energy Conversion and Management*, 50(5):1172–1179, 2009.

[125] A. Sharma, V. V. Tyagi, C. R. Chen, and D. Buddhi. Review on thermal energy storage with phase change materials and applications. *Renewable and Sustainable Energy Reviews*, 13(2):318–345, 2009.

[126] H. Li and J. Tan. An ultra-low-power medium access control protocol for body sensor network, in *27th Annual International Conference of the IEEE Engineering in Medicine and Biology Society*, pages 2451–2454, 2005. IEEE.

[127] S. Ullah, P. Khan, Y.-W. Choi, H.-S. Lee, and K. S. Kwak. MAC hurdles in body sensor networks, in *ICACT '09: Proceedings of the 11th International Conference on Advanced Communication Technology*, pages 1151–1155, Piscataway, NJ, 2009. IEEE.

[128] R. Bianchini and R. Rajamony. Power and energy management for server systems. *Computer*, 37(11):68–76, Nov. 2004.

[129] S. Roundy, E. S. Leland, J. Baker *et al.* Improving power output for vibration-based energy scavengers. *IEEE Pervasive Computing*, 4(1):28–36, 2005.

[130] 8 most "eco-friendly" Nokia mobile phones. `http://www.environmentteam.com/2010/04/07/8-most-eco-friendly-nokia-mobile-phones/`.

[131] Eco gadgets: Recyclable paper laptop for sustainable computing. `http://www.ecofriend.org/entry/eco-gadgets-recyclable-paper-laptop-for-sustainable-computing/`.

[132] L. Yang, R. Vyas, A. Rida, J. Pan, and M. M. Tentzeris. Wearable RFID-enabled sensor nodes for biomedical applications, in *Proceedings of the 2008 Electronic Components and Technology Conference*, pages 2156–2159, 2008. IEEE.

[133] G. Park, T. Rosing, M. D. Todd, C. R. Farrar, and W. Hodgkiss. Energy harvesting for structural health monitoring sensor networks. *ASCE Journal of Infrastructure Systems*, 14(1):64–79, 2008.

[134] A. Kansal, J. Hsu, M. Srivastava, and V. Raghunathan. Harvesting aware power management for sensor networks, in *43rd ACM/IEEE Design Automation Conference*, pages 651–656, 2006. ACM/IEEE.

[135] R. A. Robergs and R. Landwehr. The surprising history of the $HR_{max} = 220 - age$ equation. *Journal of Exercise Physiology*, 5(2):1–10, 2002.

[136] V. Jones, V. Gay, and P. Leijdekkers. Body sensor networks for mobile health monitoring: experience in Europe and Australia, Technical report TR-CTIT-09-43, Centre for Telematics and Information Technology, University of Twente, Enschede, 2009.

[137] K. K. Venkatasubramanian, A. Banerjee, and S. K. S. Gupta. Plethysmogram-based secure inter-sensor communication in body area networks, in *Military Communications Conference, 2008. MILCOM 2008*, pages 1–7, 2008. IEEE.

[138] D. Ajaya, J. Adarsh, S. Srinivas *et al.* Power efficiency analysis and SW development recommendations for Intel Atom based MID platforms, in *White Paper*. Intel Software Group, 2009.

[139] H. Ghasemzadeh, V. Loseu, E. Guenterberg, and R. Jafari. Sport training using body sensor networks: a statistical approach to measure wrist rotation for golf swing, in *Proceedings of the International Conference on Body Area Networks*, pages 1–8, 2009. ICST.

[140] N. Lewis. Toward cost-effective solar energy use. *Science*, 315(5813):798–801, 2007.

[141] T. Mukherjee, A. Banerjee, G. Varsamopoalos, S. K. S. Gupta, and S. Rungta. Spatio-temporal thermal-aware job scheduling to minimize energy consumption in virtualized heterogeneous data centers. *Computer Networks*, 53(17):2888–2904, June 2009.

[142] R. Burchfield and S. Venkatesan. A framework for golf training using low-cost inertial sensors, in *International Workshop on Wearable and Implantable Body Sensor Networks*, pages 267–272, 2010.

[143] P. Mistry, P. Maes, and L. Chang. Wuw – wear ur world: a wearable gestural interface, in *CHI EA '09: Proceedings of the 27th International Conference on Human Factors in Computing Systems*, pages 4111–4116, New York, NY, 2009. ACM.

[144] E. I. Gaura, J. Brusey, J. Kemp, and C. D. Thake. Increasing safety of bomb disposal missions: a body sensor network approach. *IEEE Transactions on Systems, Man and Cybernetics Part C*, 39:621–636, Nov. 2009.

[145] Shimmer 2R Platform Specifications, 2010. `http://www.shimmer-research.com/p/products/sensor-units-and-modules/shimmer-wireless-sensor-unitplatform`.

[146] A. Barth, M. Hanson, H. Powell, and J. Lach. Tempo 3.1: a body area sensor network platform for continuous movement assessment, in *Sixth International Workshop on Wearable and Implantable Body Sensor Networks*, pages 71–76, Berkeley, CA, 2009. IEEE.

[147] BSN node v3 Specifications, `http://ubimon.doc.ic.ac.uk/bsn/a1875.html`, 2009.

[148] TelosB mote specifications. `http://www.xbow.com/Products/Product_pdf_files/Wireless_pdf/TelosB_Datasheet.pdf`, 2006.

[149] Imote2 platform specifications. `http://www.xbow.com/Products/Product_pdf_files/Wireless_pdf/Imote2_Datasheet.pdf`, 2008.

[150] S. Nabar, A. Banerjee, S. K. S. Gupta, and R. Poovendran. Evaluation of body sensor network platforms: a design space and benchmarking analysis, in *Wireless Health 2010*, WH '10, pages 118–127, New York, NY, 2010. ACM.

[151] X. Chen, A. Waluyo, I. Pek, and W.-S. Yeoh. Mobile middleware for wireless body area network, in *Engineering in Medicine and Biology Society (EMBC), 2010 Annual International Conference of the IEEE*, pages 5504–5507, 2010. IEEE.

[152] G. Fortino, A. Guerrieri, F. Bellifemine, and R. Giannantonio. Spine2: developing BSN applications on heterogeneous sensor nodes, in *IEEE International Symposium on Industrial Embedded Systems, 2009. SIES '09*, pages 128–131, 2009.

[153] M. Mozumdar, F. Gregoretti, L. Lavagno, L. Vanzago, and S. Olivieri. A framework for modeling, simulation and automatic code generation of sensor network application, in *5th Annual IEEE Communications Society Conference on Sensor, Mesh and Ad Hoc Communications and Networks, 2008. SECON '08*, pages 515–522, 2008. IEEE.

[154] J. B. Lim, B. Jang, S. Yoon, M. L. Sichitiu, and A. G. Dean. Raptex: rapid prototyping tool for embedded communication systems. *ACM Transactions on Sensors and Networks*, 7(7):1–40, Aug. 2010.

[155] E. Cheong, E. A. Lee, and Y. Zhao. Viptos: a graphical development and simulation environment for TinyoS-based wireless sensor networks, in *Proceedings of the 3rd International Conference on Embedded Networked Sensor Systems, SenSys '05*, page 302, New York, NY, 2005. ACM.

[156] W. P. McCartney and N. Sridhar. Tosdev: a rapid development environment for TinyOS, in *Proceedings of the 4th International Conference on Embedded Networked Sensor Systems, SenSys '06*, pages 387–388, New York, NY, 2006. ACM.

Index

ACM MSWiM, 127
active attack, 64
actuation, 20
AES, 34
aggregate effects, 31
air flow rate, 43
Android, 106
anesthesia, 21
antenna, 13
    chip antenna, 13
    inverted-F antenna, 13
    surface-mount antenna, 13
architectural model, 43
Architecture Analysis and Design Language
    (AADL), 41
assistive devices, 9
assurance cases, 34
asymmetric crypto-systems, 66
asymmetric-key cryptography, 68
authentication, 63
authorization, 63
availability, 63

BAN, 6, 36
BAN-CPS, 45
BAN safety approaches, 37
BAND-AiDe, 42
base station, 10
binary point, 111
biochannel, 14
biometrics, 71
biosensors, 5
blood pressure, 5
Bluetooth, 104
body area network, 9
bolus, 20
broadcast receiver, 107
BSN, 6
BSNBench, 115

car area network (CAN), 15
cell-phone, 11
Central Drugs Standard Control Organisation
    (CDSCO), 33

chaff points, 75
channel model, 14
    log-normal, 14
    Rayleigh, 14
    Ricean, 14
code safety, 38
communication protocol stack, 12
    application framework, 13
    application support sublayer, 13
    medium access control (MAC), 13
    network layer, 13
    physical layer, 13
computing power management, 87
computing properties, 43
conference, 127
    ACM Wireless Health, 127
    IEEE BSN, 127
    IEEE EMBC, 127
    IEEE Infocom, 127
    IEEE Milcom, 127
    Percom, 127
control system safety, 38
coprocessor, 113
critical events, 37
criticality, 37
cryptography, 68
cyber-physical, 4, 30
cyber-physical security, 65
cyber-physical systems, 42
cycle life, 16

data confidentiality, 63
data integrity, 63
denial of service, 64
design-space determination, 114
design-space exploration, 114
differential equations, 18
distinctiveness, 71
duty cycling, 88

eavesdropping, 63
ECG, 112
electrocardiogram, 5
electromyogram, 5

electronic health records (EHRs), 3
electronic medical records (EMRs), 3
electronic patient records (EPRs), 3
embedded system, 10
energy-efficiency, 18
energy harvesting, 88
energy-neutral, 88
energy-storage devices, 85
energy-sustainability, 84
errors, 14
    burst errors, 14
    fading errors, 14
    random bit errors, 14
European Committee for Electrotechnical
        Standardization (Cenelec), 33
European Committee for Standardization (CEN), 33
event-driven, 15

fast charging time, 16
fast Fourier transform, 19
FDA, 21
FFT, 112
FIFO, 106
filters, 18
flash memory, 112
flexible electronics, 11
floating point, 109
Food and Drug Administration (FDA), 39
form factor, 113
formal models, 39
FPGA, 113
fuzzy vault, 74

galvanic skin response, 5
GCPS, 42
GeM-REM, 18
generative models, 17
generic infusion pump, 38
gravimetric energy density, 16
green energy sources, 84

HAL, 106
harvesting theory, 88
health information exchange (HIE), 4
healthcare, 1
heat transferred, 43
heterogeneous, 10
HIL, 106
HIPAA, 64
Holter monitors, 9
hospital, 9
HPL, 105
humidity, 22
hybrid automata, 61

IEEE task group 6 (TG6), 10
IEEE TG6 standard, 11

implanted, 9, 11
in-vivo, 14
industry, 11
    Apple, 15
    Atmel, 11
    Google, 15
    Intel, 11
    Texas Instruments, 11
    Windows, 15
infusion pump, 38
infusion rate, 43
intended interactions, 31
intensive-care unit (ICU), 9
intent receivers, 107
intentional interactions, 42
interaction safety, 38
Internet-of-things, 65
inverted-F antenna, 113

journal, 127
    ACM TECS, 127
    ACM TOSN, 127
    IEEE Proceedings, 127
    IEEE TITB, 127
    IEEE TON, 127

key distribution, 68
    asymmetric cryptography-based, 69
    communication-based, 69
    solely pre-deployment-based, 68

Lagrangian interpolation, 76
LCPS, 43
local CPSes (LCPSes), 43
long-range communication, 14

MAC protocol, 14
    carrier sense multiple access-collision avoidance
        (CSMA-CA), 14
    frequency-hopping spread spectrum (FHSS), 14
man-in-the-middle, 64
master-key-based key-distribution schemes, 66
master–slave connection, 14
medical device, 11, 33
    camera pill, 11
    class I, 33
    class II, 33
    class III, 33
    greater risk, 35
    infusion pump, 11
    minimal risk, 35
    pulse oximeter, 9
medical device data systems (MDDSes), 34
medical device networks (MDNs), 9
medical devices, 36
medical facility, 24
mesh networking, 14

micro-controller, 105
microprocessor, 113
middleware, 23
mission-critical, 29
mobility model, 91
   Lévy-walk model, 91
   random-way-point, 91
model analysis, 40
model checking, 44
model development, 40
model-based engineering (MBE), 40
model-predictive control system, 38
modeling constructs, 44
monitored parameter, 43
morphology, 18
motes, 11
   BSN node v3, 13
   iMote2, 13
   Mica2, 13
   Shimmer, 13
   TelosB, 13
multi-hop, 11
MyHeart, 6

National Institutes for Health (NIH), 127
National Science Foundation (NSF), 127
near-field communication (NFC), 14
network safety, 37

onCreate, 108
operating system, 15
overcharge tolerance, 16
overhearing, 14

pacemakers, 39
Pacific Bridge Medical, 33
packet-drop ratio (PDR), 13
passive attack, 63
patient, 36
patient safety, 36
patient-centric, 3
peak detection, 112
Pennes' bioheat equation, 43, 56
personal area networks (PANs), 9
personal computing, 9
pervasive care system, 5
   Ayushman, 5
   Code-Blue, 5
   HealthGear, 5
   Lifeshirt, 5
   Microcompaq, 5
   MyHeart, 5
   SenseWear, 5
   UbiMon, 5
pervasive health-monitoring system, 1, 26
pervasive healthcare, 2
pharmacokinetic model, 21

photoplethysmogram, 5
physical dynamics, 43
physical environment, 36
physical properties, 43
physiological-signal-based key agreement
   feature generation, 74
   polynomial choice, 75
   PSKA, 70
   vault acknowledgment, 76
   vault creation, 75
   vault exchange, 75
   vault locking, 75
   vault unlocking, 76
post-operative, 9
pre-deployment, 69
privacy, 64
proactive, 3
probabilistic key-distribution schemes, 66
processor, 11
   application-specific integrated circuit (ASIC), 11
   ARM, 11
   ATMEGA 128, 11
   field-programmable gate array (FPGA), 11
   hybrid platforms, 11
   Intel Atom, 11
   MSP430, 11
   xScale, 11
processor frequency scaling, 92
pulse oximeter, 39

radio, 14
   6lowPAN, 14
   Bluetooth, 14
   Bluetooth low-power, 14
   ZigBee, 14
radio sleep scheduling, 92
RAM, 112
reception, 13
region boundary, 43
region of impact (ROIm), 43
region of interest (ROIn), 43
reliable, 11
research groups, 127
   Center for Wireless Health, 127
   ESSP Lab, 127
   Harvard Sensor Networks Lab, 127
   IMPACT Lab at Arizona State University, 127
   Imperial College London, 127
   Media Labs, 127
   NSL at the University of Washington, 127
   UAV Center for Wireless Health, 127
   Wireless Life Sciences Alliances, 127
retina prosthesis, 9

safety, 36
SAR, 56
scavenging, 87

scenario safety, 37
security, 63
   accountability, 34
   availability, 34
   confidentiality, 34
   integrity, 34
self-discharge rate, 16
sensor, 10
   ECG patches, 11
   humidity, 11
   light, 11
   nanosensors, 11
   smart clothing, 11
   temperature, 11
signal correlation, 112
signal repositories, 118
   Berlin Database of Emotional Speech (EmoDB), 118
   CASIA Gait Database, 118
   Consolidated Human Activity Database, 118
   Impact database, 118
   MIT BIH Physiobank, 118
   UC Irvine EEG database, 118
single-hop, 10
skin temperature, 5
smart phones, 2, 9
SmartVest, 6
social media, 15
   Facebook, 15
   MySpace, 15
software, 15
   Android, 15
   iOS, 15
   iPhone, 15
   SilverLight, 15
software engineering, 40
   software testing, 39
   software verification, 39
software safety, 38
spatio-temporal cyber-physical interactions, 42
spatio-temporal distribution of operation, 86

spatio-temporal hybrid automata (STHA), 60
spatio-temporal partial differential equations, 60
specific absorption rate, 56
specific heat, 43
spoofing, 63
State Food and Drug Administration (SFDA), 33
stochastic models, 88
surface-mount antenna, 113
sustainability, 84
sustainable BAN software, 89
sustainable computing platforms, 87

telemedicine, 2
temperature, 22
temperature rise, 43
temporal variance, 71
TinyOS, 19, 106
topographic specificity, 72
transmission, 13
TunnelCreek platform, 114

un-intentional interactions, 42
unintended interactions, 31
universal asynchronous receiver/transmitter (UART), 106
unobtrusive, 9
usability, 6, 70

wave-dipole antenna, 13
wearability, 13
wearable, 11
Wifi protected access, 66
windkessel, 18
wireless channel, 14
wireless PANs (WPANs), 9
wireless sensor networks (WSNs), 9
WPA, 66
WPA2, 66

ZigBee, 104